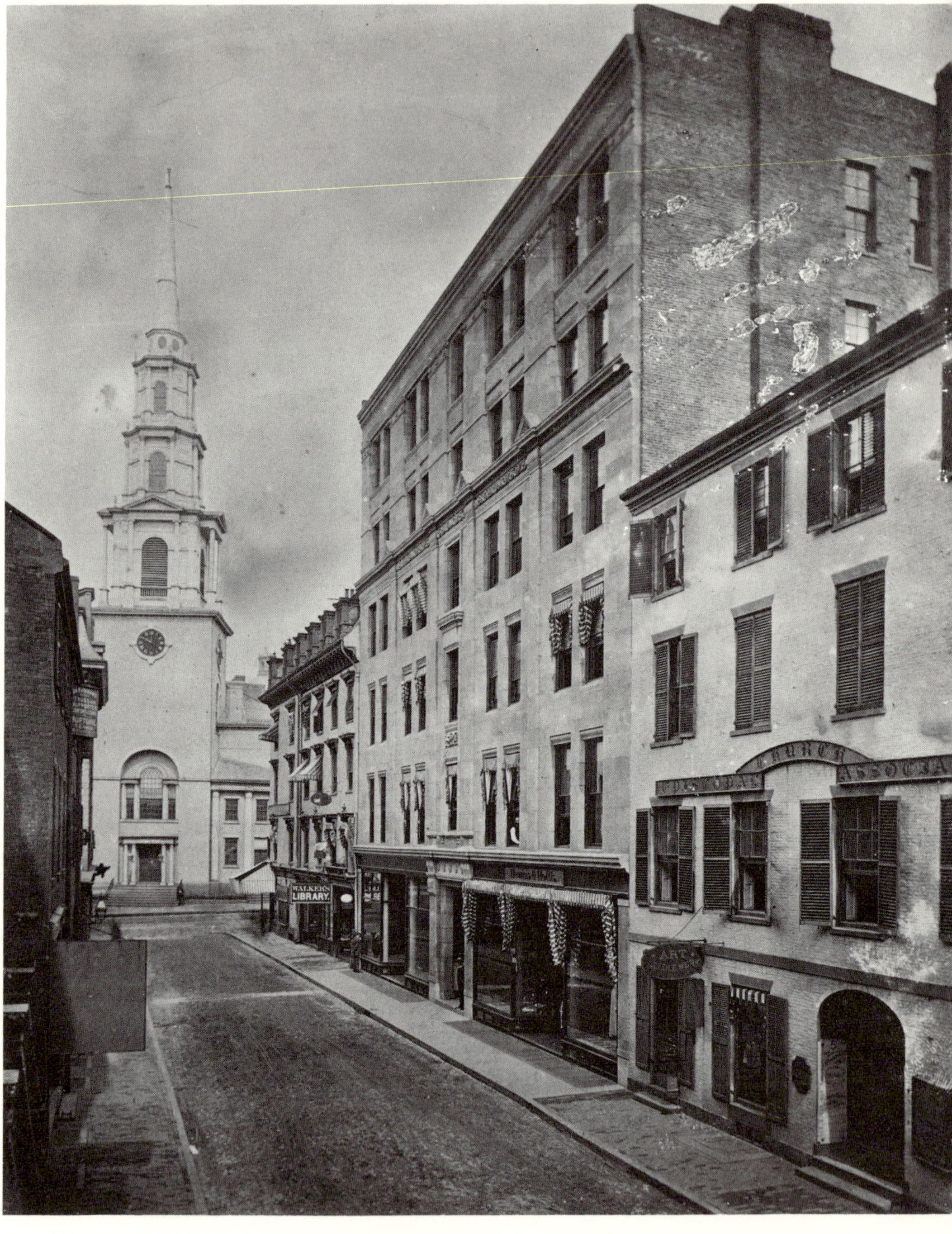

Hamilton Place, about 1885.
The Library's first rooms at number 5
were on ground floor through arched door at right.
Park Street Church in background.

The Centennial History of the Boston Medical Library 1875 • 1975

Joseph E. Garland

The Boston Medical Library
in the Francis A. Countway
Library of Medicine

Boston 1975

In Memoriam

JOSEPH GARLAND

1893 - 1973

MIRA CROWELL GARLAND

1896 - 1974

CONTENTS

Chronology

1800—Ward Nicholas Boylston gives Boylston Medical Library to Harvard.

1803—Boston Society for Medical Improvement organized.

July 1, 1805—First Boston Medical Library (Second Social Library) founded by John Collins Warren, James Jackson and members of the Medical Improvement Society.

May 3, 1826—Boston Medical Library ceded to Boston Athenaeum.

1835—Boston Society for Medical Observation organized.

December 21, 1874—Six members of Observation Society meet in office of Henry Ingersoll Bowditch to organize Boston Medical Library Association.

August 20, 1875—Boston Medical Library Association formally organized. Oliver Wendell Holmes president, James Read Chadwick librarian, Edwin H. Brigham assistant librarian.

October 18, 1875—Library opens at 5 Hamilton Place.

December 3, 1878—New quarters at 19 Boylston Place dedicated.

November 1879—Directory for Nurses, first in U.S., opens at BML.

1888—Dr. Holmes resigns presidency and presents his library to BML.

October 24, 1892—James Francis Ballard begins work as stack boy.

October 7, 1894—Dr. Holmes dies.

January 12, 1901—New library building at 8 The Fenway dedicated.

1901-1904—Academy of Medicine proposed and deposed.

1904—Mrs. Sarah E. Potter bequeaths $150,000 for Warren B. Potter Memorial.

September 23, 1905—Dr. Chadwick dies. Succeeded as librarian by John Woodford Farlow.

1918—Librarian Farlow publishes *The History of the Boston Medical Library*; Assistant Librarian Ballard publishes first edition of BML Medical Classification, later widely adopted.

1919-1921—Union with Harvard Medical School Library under discussion.

1921—Boston Medical History Club organized under auspices of BML, Harvey Cushing first president.

1924-1926—Academy of Medicine exhumed and reinterred.

1928—Dr. Farlow retires, succeeded by Charles Fairbank Painter; Ballard appointed Director; joint fund drive launched with Massachusetts Medical Society.

1930—Shell of stack addition built and occupied by the Medical Society and *The New England Journal of Medicine.*

1931—Dr. William Norton Bullard bequeaths his collection of medical incunabula.

1938—Dr. Painter retires as librarian, succeeded by Henry Rouse Viets.

1941—Carnegie (Fleming) Survey recommends BML concentrate on regional reference services.

1947—Affiliation with Massachusetts Medical Society increases dues income by 70 per cent; Metcalf Plan of improvement undertaken.

1952—Beckwith Report urges modernization and capital fund campaign.

1953-1954—Boston Medical Library Greater Service Program raises $316,000; stacks installed in wing and other alterations completed.

May 14, 1955—Director Ballard dies after 63 years with BML.

1956—Charles C. Colby 3rd appointed librarian, Dr. Viets curator.

December 9, 1958—President Howard B. Sprague proposes union with Harvard Medical Library being planned by Dean George Packer Berry.

January 1960—BML President Sprague and Harvard President Nathan M. Pusey sign agreement to unite in the Francis A. Countway Library of Medicine.

1962—Dr. Beth Vincent bequeaths BML $100,000.

May 12, 1964—Cornerstone of Countway Library laid.

June 16, 1965—Countway opens for business; BML vacates 8 The Fenway, purchased by Boston Conservatory of Music; Ralph T. Esterquest is first librarian of Countway, Mr. Colby first associate librarian for BML Services.

1966—Countway Associates founded in behalf of Rare Books Collection.

1967—Countway Library carries on BML's regional role as New England Regional Medical Library for the National Library of Medicine.

August 10, 1968—Librarian Esterquest dies, succeeded by his assistant, Harold Bloomquist.

July 5, 1969—Dr. Viets dies.

1970—BML receives bequest of $1,078,600 from estate of Dennistoun M. Bell.

1971—Massachusetts Medical Society doubles its dues to the BML from five to ten dollars per capita.

1973—Oliver Wendell Holmes Endowment for Rare Books Department launched.

Preface

The opportunity to chronicle the history of *any* medical library, not to mention that of the most distinguished in the Western Hemisphere, knocks almost less than infrequently at the humble door of the professional writer. When it does, the rap has a gauntlet ring to it. And indeed, President Bentley P. Colcock challenged me (graciously, without laying it too heavily upon my laymanship) to come up with "a vitalizing and stimulating human record of great men and a great work" for the centennial of what he was pleased to call "an extraordinary institution."

At the time I felt in no position either to agree or demur, having more than once some years earlier shouldered my gingerly way through the overflowing dust bins up to the, shall I say, *unruffled* upper levels of the old library at 8 The Fenway, and once having even shaken the young hand of old Ballard, eyeing me quizzically from behind his barricade of books.

So I concluded to test a lance against this *bibliotheca medica,* as the formidable Latinist would have it, whose great cumbersome front portal, I would learn, was by itself enough to frighten away all but the most case-hardened of Beacon Street's medical secretaries. The fact is that by 1973 I had so succeeded in shedding the psychic burden of three successive medical progenitors that I had discovered the strength to stand by my decision to do this book in the face not only of my revered father's approbation, but of the faintly nepotistical coincidence that he was my subject's immediate past president.

As it turned out (and will appear, I hope), the enthusiasm of Bentley Colcock and his persuasive emissaries, Charles H. Bradford and Jean A. Curran, for the grimy old place proved out in spades, as they say. I learned that the Boston Medical Library *is* an extraordinary institution, the great work of several generations of men, some of them great, all of them dedicated to the ideals of their profeession and to the joys of literature and the arts. And it is not too much to say that its longevity and continuing vitality through an existence which spans nearly two centuries (including a few years of suspended animation) have been passed from preceptor to pupil by those thorough masters of their calling whose mark is in having added the graceful and leavening influence of learning—as Dr. Holmes put it and did it—to their natural gifts.

That mark today seals the somehow equal, yet somehow separate, union of the Library with its childhood sweetheart, the Medical School of Harvard University.

The construction of this work would have been much more difficult on anything less solid than the 1918 foundation of Dr. Farlow's *History,* and much less interesting without the "Medical Library Notes" which it amused him to leave behind. Helpful adjuncts were the meticulous *History of the Massachusetts Medical Society* published five years later by its and the BML's faithful Secretary, Dr. Walter L. Burrage, and Dr. Thomas F. Harrington's *History of the Harvard Medical School* of 1905.

For their assistance, contributions and cooperation in the research stage I am grateful to Charles C. Colby 3rd; Richard J. Wolfe, Mrs. Willa Folch-Pi and the rest of the Rare Books staff; Dr. James M. Faulkner; Miss Dorothy Murphy, Emerita of the Harvard Medical Alumni Association office; Professor John P. Coolidge; and Harold Bloomquist and his co-workers at the Francis A. Countway Library of Medicine. The manuscript owes its substantial improvement to the comments of Doctors Lloyd E. Hawes, Robert W. Buck, Curran and Bradford, and of Librarians Bloomquist, Colby and Wolfe. To President Hawes and Mr. Wolfe I am further indebted for their help in guiding the finished creation through the press, as I am, always, to R.C.G. for guiding *me* from the start.

Joseph E. Garland

Gloucester, Massachusetts
March 1975

Introduction

At the ripe age of one hundred, the Boston Medical Library publishes this book of its beginnings, its growth, its several homes and the succession of librarians and doctors who have constantly extended the "growing edge" of the Library into the unknown future. Author Joseph E. Garland (Harvard A.B.) is well known for his histories of the North Shore of Massachusetts Bay and of two Boston hospitals. For the present work, he has chosen the style of a well-researched raconteur; each chapter covers a period of change either in the purposes of the Library, its physical plant, or its leadership. He reveals periods of expansion, but also periods of stalemate due to frustration and lack of an ongoing purpose. The Library has been haunted on many occasions by the specter of too many books for the available stacks; it has chronically suffered from the "cup runneth over" syndrome. For many years one librarian with one or two assistants ran the details of daily acquisitions, cataloging, etc. Garland tells not merely how Topsy grew, but why she grew, and by her very nature, must continue to grow.

A hundredth birthday is a wonderful thing. When a human reaches the age of 80, 85 or 90, we stand amazed at the ability of some of these to show extraordinary vitality, a ripe knowledge of things past, and a maturity in response to things present. We note a certain mellowing of personality, a slowing of pace, and a lessened push to conquer the world. But this is the reaction of humans, not of institutions. On attaining the age of one hundred, a human is only a shadow of himself both mentally and physically. Institutions cannot be equated on this human scale. Many governments and religions have survived with vigor for centuries, yes even for millenia. We know this is not usually true. The alphabet soup of governmental agencies staggers our memory by their short lives. What did C.C.C. stand for anyway in the 1930s?

Entering its one hundred and first year, the Library, after a decade of marriage with the Harvard Medical Library, lives in an architecturally stunning and highly functional home, the Countway Library of Medicine. It still has space for new gifts of books and archives. However, the footage of empty shelves dwindles daily. The recently printed multivolume catalog of the Countway holdings soon will require additional volumes to list new acquisitions. The main index catalogs are supplemented by the addition of new cards once, even twice daily. Serving New England's medical public has become big business.

At one hundred and one, the Library does not doze away. It not only remains wide awake, responding to new demands for new services, but in the past decade it has taken on new vigor. In reaction to the dwindling supply of public monies which have helped to maintain its very existence, the Library has organized the Oliver Wendell Holmes Endowment Fund as a means of raising private capital from public-spirited donors for future sustenance. Its social and meeting rooms on the fifth floor are constantly used by both physicians and surrounding community organizations. These are continuing and visible evidences of the Library's ability to change, to become creative in an accelerating fashion, and to show that it has found Ponce de León's fountain of youth to continually meet the demands of today's medical profession. The Library cannot celebrate its Centennial; WE do. In 1975, as in former years, scores of men and women supply the elixir of youth to the Library. But these same men and women realize that they will someday have to withdraw from the scene, and must recruit younger people who will dedicate themselves to guide the Library for the next decade, for the next century, and yea, perhaps even for centuries.

The Trustees join me in praising Mr. Garland's splendid and readable book, a striking tribute to our beloved Library!

Lloyd E. Hawes, M.D.
President
Boston Medical Library

The Centennial History of the Boston Medical Library

1875

·

1975

1

A Diminutive Commencement

1805 · 1826

A physician of common sense without erudition is better than a learned one without common sense, but the thorough master of his profession must have learning added to his natural gifts.

Dr. Oliver Wendell Holmes, at the dedication of the new quarters of the Boston Medical Library on December 3, 1878.

The Autocrat was not unmindful, of course, that his hearers had chosen him the first president of their reincarnated medical library precisely because they considered him the *ne plus ultra* of his third category. "What illuminates a country like its scholarship?" he declaimed pleasantly, "and what is the nest that hatches scholars but a library?"

The first discernible nesting effort aimed at hatching medical scholars appears to have occurred 130 years before Harvard's anatomist and man of letters cast these dedicatory aphorisms among his colleagues in medicine and learning. At that distant time, erudition was on the whole absent from the armamentarium of the practitioner, while common sense—judging from the known results of clinical intervention—was hardly less so. It did not matter greatly that there was no seat of academic medical education anywhere in the Western Hemisphere.

The year was 1748. By the Treaty of Aix-la-Chapelle George II gained some brief respite from England's enemies in Europe and the colonies which the royal physician, Dr. Richard Mead, took advantage of to send across the Atlantic Harvard College's first recorded acquisition of medical literature, his *Mechanical Account of Poisons,* 1702, and his *Medica sacra, sive de morbis insignioribus qui in bibliis memorantur commentarius,* just published. The same year William Vassall donated "Twelve Tables of the Human Bones, finely engraved, framed," by the contemporary German anatomist, Bernhard Siegfried Albinus; a human skeleton was received from Francis Archibald, and William Davis gave the college a collection of wax-filled blood vessels.

The moving spirit behind this ghostly library-cabinet may have been

John Winthrop, the second Hollis Professor of Mathematics and Natural Philosophy, and the most inquisitive scientific mind in New England. Winthrop was thirty-three. Two years previously he had set up the first laboratory of experimental physics in the New York. The professor was an energetic and eclectic collector in the natural sciences, just the man to interest himself in skeletons, venae stuffed with wax, and treatises on poison. In 1750 Davis added more anatomical preparations. William James of the island of Jamaica shipped up a set of "the most approved Medical Authors" and twenty-five pounds in cash in 1752, and in 1758 that interesting merchant of Boston, James Bowdoin, provided a microscope. Also about this time, the college's skeleton force was doubled.

The nest for what bid fair to be America's first medical school rose up in smoke on the night of January 24, 1764. The smallpox had invaded Boston, and the General Court of Massachusetts fled across the Charles River to reconvene in Harvard Hall while the students vacationed. A spark, a flame. . . and hall, library and the most approved medical authors, the anatomical tables, the waxy curiosities and the bony couple were in ashes. Lamented the *Boston Post-Boy and Advertiser*: "This Collection would have been very serviceable to a Professor of Physic and Anatomy, when the revenues of the College should have been sufficient to subsist a gentleman in this character."

By Harvard's fire the library of the Pennsylvania Hospital, founded in 1760, came into the precedence. In 1765 the College of Philadelphia initiated formal academic medical instruction in the colonies. Harvard had to rest content with organizing the first post-Revolution medical department at the hands of Dr. John Warren in 1782. It was the idea of the new president, Joseph Willard, who had been diverted from medicine into the ministry when he was young and impressionable, which probably accounts for his excitement upon attending a sequel to the anatomical lectures which Continental Surgeon Warren had given in the Boston military hospital toward the end of the war.

For the benefit of the medical department which President Willard proposed in 1782, he hoped that the library of Harvard *University* (as it had been called since 1780) would be "enriched with a collection of the approved authors in anatomy, surgery, physic, chemistry, etc. . . a collection more perfect than any in America, as soon as circumstances will permit." They did not. The small medical faculty, and indeed the "university,"were hard pressed to keep alive after the General Court cut off Harvard's financial support forever in 1786 in a tiff with Willard over his

Federalist politics. And there is no evidence that anything more than an odd volume ever arose from the ashes of 1764.

Instead, such meagre surplus of medical scholarship as could be spared from the private collections of physicians appears to have gravitated to the Massachusetts Medical Society, which the year after its chartering in 1781 resolved to have a library of its own and put Dr. Aaron Dexter in charge of the project. By 1788 the titles on its shelf in his home on Milk Street had crept along to the sum of twenty-six, principally by courtesy of Dr. James Lloyd, who had the distinction of having taken a course in obstetrics at Guy's Hospital in London. Lloyd's real mark on posterity, however, is his preceptorship of Dr. Joseph Warren, the charismatic, enigmatic patriot who passed the lamp along to his worshipping younger brother, John, before spilling out his life in the hot dust of Breed's, erroneously known as Bunker, Hill on the heights of Charlestown.

But although Dexter was the first Professor of Chemistry and Materia Medica, and the volumes of the Society in his care were presumably available to the faculty of the undernourished infant medical school, the students were across the Charles in Cambridge, shivering through lectures and demonstrations in the basement of the rebuilt Harvard Hall.

Happily for President Willard, the wished-for enrichment of his medical school's library arrived as another transatlantic transplant while he was still in office to congratulate himself and the university's benefactor, Ward Nicholas Boylston, né Ward Hallowell.

When Hallowell reached twenty-one in 1770 he had adopted the name of his maternal uncle, Nicholas Boylston, an act of affection which suggests that that eminent Boston merchant already had adopted *him*. Ward traveled Europe, settled in London and secured his fortune. In 1800 he turned homeward, philanthropically inclined and desirous of memorializing his mother's family. Uncle Nicholas had made a start in 1771 by endowing the professorship in rhetoric and oratory at Harvard which bears his name, fifty years exactly after Ward's Great-Uncle Zabdiel Boylston introduced inoculation for smallpox to America.

For his part, upon arriving home in Boston in 1800, Ward Boylston gave the medical school in the inoculator's name some 1100 volumes of selected authors assembled mainly by Dr. John Nichols of London, and a number of anatomical plates and preparations of John's father, Francis Nichols, late Professor of Anatomy at Oxford. Further, he provided annuities for additional accessions and for an annual Boylston prize essay in medicine, and presented to the Boylston Medical Library (as it became officially in 1803)—among other family portraits by John Singleton Copley—the luxuriously robed figure of Uncle Nicholas, shrewd of visage, shorn and capped, which hangs in the entrance court of the Francis A. Countway Library of Medicine.[1]

A score of years after the opening of its medical department Harvard at last had a proper collection of the approved authors. But if it was adequate to the times, it was miserably out of place. School, library and students impracticably were in Cambridge, while the faculty and most of the profession resided eight miles away by wretched road in Boston. The construction of Cambridge Bridge for toll traffiic in 1793 reduced the distance, but not significantly.

Possibly Harvard's incorporation, seemingly forever, of Boylston's handsome gift of books within the college library served to push a small group of mostly younger physicians and surgeons, across the river in Boston, to organize the Society for Medical Improvement. Their object was to convene Thursday evenings to present and discuss papers, and to gather a library of their own in the home of Dr. John Fleet in Milk Street. Their participation in this enterprise was the first known collaboration of those two lifelong friends who would change the course of American medicine, James Jackson and John Collins Warren, son of John Warren. Both of them foresaw that since the patients, as objects of profit and pedagogy, and the practitioners and preceptors, were nearly all in Boston, and since Boston could not easily move to Cambridge, then Harvard's medical school must one day move to Boston.

James Jackson in 1803 was twenty-six. After his graduation from Harvard College, where he first met Warren, he studied abroad with Sir Astley Cooper at Guy's and others and returned to Boston to share in introducing Edward Jenner's vaccination to America almost on the heels of Benjamin Waterhouse, his medical school mentor. It was a brilliant opening to a career which elicited the veneration of Holmes, who remembered Dr. Jackson as "a pure and noble character. . . of serenely cheerful aspect, pleasant, inspiriting manner, always neatly and plainly dressed, exact in all his habits, punctual as the morning sun, searching in his inquiries and examinations, precise to minuteness in his directions, full of the sober wisdom of experience, but always open to new convictions. . ."[2]

John Collins Warren at the founding of the Society for Medical Improvement in 1803 was twenty-five. Like Jackson, he had studied with Cooper in London and had just returned to enter into partnership with his father and assist him with dissections in his course on anatomy and surgery in Cambridge. He would succeed to the Harvard chair on John

Warren's death in 1815, and would be followed in turn after thirty-two more years by Holmes, to whom the younger Warren was the greatest surgeon of his day in America. "A spare man," wrote Dr. Holmes of John Collins Warren, "with strongly marked features, of austere expression, authoritative manners, sometimes careless, occasionally aiming at elegance in personal presentment. . . He was one of the best educated medical men of his generation among us. . . He commanded allegiance and obedience where Dr. Jackson inspired love and confidence. . . always deliberate, always cool, with a grim smile in sudden emergencies where weaker men would have looked perplexed and wiped their foreheads."[3]

Jackson and Warren were joined in their Medical Improvement Society by John Dixwell, twenty-six, bachelor of medicine from Harvard in 1800, and John Clarke Howard, thirty, who also had studied abroad after his apprenticeship to Dr. Samuel Danforth of Boston, *Old Danfurt*. . . Howard, beloved by all, "whose tender sympathy and unwearied attention," in the admiring words of James Thacher, "evinced that he had not failed to profit by his own experience of the sufferings incident to feebleness and disease," who would live only seven more years.[4] Youngest was George Cheyne Shattuck, first of the medical Shattucks, a mere twenty, fresh out of Dartmouth and four years to go for his Pennsylvania medical degree. . . an impressive lad to gain admittance to such a company.

Beside these were three whose ages climbed up to the fifty-nine years of John Jeffries. *Doctor Jeffers* learned medicine and loyalty to George III from James Lloyd. His fame arose with his experiments during a brace of bold balloon ascents in Europe soon after the Revolution, augurs of the science of space. Dr. Holmes dimly recalled him. "He came, probably, to administer the professional *coup de grace* to an aged relative of my own, who had been given up by his attending physician, and only awaited the final word of a skilled and ancient expert to authorize his departing in peace."[5] Seventh was John Homans, fifty or so, like all save Shattuck a Harvard graduate, veteran of the bloody surgery of the Revolution, and like Warren and Shattuck, medical progenitor.

Finally, there was the Improvement Society's librarian, John Fleet, thirty-seven, co-member with George Holmes Hall of the Harvard Medical School's first graduating class in 1788, first assistant appointed, in 1793, to John Warren. Ink was his pap; his father and uncle, John and Thomas Fleet, were the Boston printers and publishers. He had succeeded to the librarianship of the Massachusetts Medical Society in 1800, when he moved its books into his Milk Street house. Unblessed with wife and family, Fleet had no ready excuse for refusing a few more feet of shelf and browsing room to the Improvement Society.[6]

Not that the two medical libraries for which he was responsible besides his own were squeezing Dr. Fleet out of house and home. All together they probably didn't amount to a tenth of the eleven hundred volumes so impossibly distant in the Boylston collection at Cambridge. Justin Winsor, librarian of the Boston Public Library and later of Harvard College, observed that the deficiencies in the libraries of the area early in the nineteenth century were such that "research was stopped in every direction by want of books;" as late as 1817, he judged, all the public and semi-public libraries in Boston and Cambridge contained no more than sixty thousand volumes, many of them duplicates.[7]

Mindful of the cultural penalties and sacrifices of revolution, the Massachusetts General Court in 1798 had passed an act enabling seven or more citizens to organize proprietary library societies, serially in each town. In 1804 the Boston bar led off with the First Social, or Social Law Library, still functioning today. The doctors then reversed the usual order and followed the lawyers. On July 1, 1805 Warren, Jackson and others in the Medical Improvement Society founded the Second Social, or Boston Medical Library. The clergy trailed with the Fourth Social, or Theological Library in 1807—the Third Social, the Scientific, having cut into line between them, probably in 1806 although the exact date is uncertain.[8]

With slight ceremony the members of the Improvement Society implanted their few books as the seed within the shell of this small oyster. Since their collection was already in the custody of John Fleet, it fell to him to be the first librarian of the Boston Medical Library. John G. Coffin was elected secretary, John Collins Warren treasurer, and James Jackson and John C. Howard trustees. The proprietors voted to assess themselves ten dollars a year, and on December 30, 1805 announced:

> The Boston Medical Library will be opened Thursday next at Dr. Fleet's. A few books only have arrived. N.B. Books received and delivered on Mondays and Thursdays between 3 and 5 P.M.

Secretary Coffin was one of the fourteen children of Pastor Paul Coffin of New Buxton, Maine. He had been practising in Boston for five years after an apprenticeship to his Uncle Charles Coffin at Newburyport in an arrangement which must have sprung from a combination of necessity and convenience. Surely he was unusually able for all his country education, for he was an attending physician and one of the board of managers of the Boston Dispensary, and in 1823 would found and edit the *Boston Medical Intelligencer*, a precursor to the *Boston*

Medical and Surgical Journal. In 1818 Coffin published *Discourses on Cold and Warm Bathing; with Remarks on the Effects of Drinking Cold Water in Warm Weather,* exulting quietly that "for many years past, during the summer, I have daily used ice in whatever I have drunk at dinner—in water, beer, cyder, etc., & this more freely as the weather has been warmer. This habit has been agreeable & refreshing."

That its founders had something more in mind than the edification of the profession in establishing a medical library in Boston is implied by J. C. Warren's concurrent commencement of a private anatomy course for medical students and physicians in rooms at 49 Marlborough Street (renamed as an extension of Washington Street in 1824), near Franklin Street, over White's apothecary. There is some suggestion here that while the corpus of Harvard's medical department remained faithfully stabled in Cambridge, the proboscis was sniffing under the tent flap across the river. The business end of the animal further insinuated itself in 1807 with the choice of Warren as successor to Fleet and the removal of the Second Social, or Boston Medical Library's growing collection to Amos Smith's apothecary at 39 Marlborough Street, a door or so away from the rump (to use the other anatomical extreme) medical school. The books were now accessible throughout the business day of Mr. Smith, who was appointed sub-librarian under the keen eye of the dissector when he wasn't rolling pills.

The first catalogue of the Boston Medical Library (they were customarily printed by the Fleets) was published promptly in 1806, with an abstract of the rules. Each proprietor was permitted to borrow as many of the forty-two volumes as he owned shares (there were twenty-nine titles) and to keep them from one to five weeks according to their size, which somehow made it follow that fines should be weighed by the same measure, from ten to twenty cents a week. Rule 6 stated that "the Sublibrarian will receive fines, but he will not undertake to demand them," a stricture which prompted one of his latter-day successors made of sterner stuff to riposte, "Query: How many fines not demanded did he receive?"[9] The nonpayment of fines entitled a proprietor to have his name posted inside the apothecary's door; the reward for three more weeks of unregenerated sin was suspension. Titles included such as Parkinson and Kinglake on gout, Cox on insanity, Cooper on cataract, Merriman and Schoolbred on vaccine, Squirrel and Moseley on cow pox, and Ring's *Answer to Moseley,* indicative of the preoccupations of the Boston profession, besides a scattering of British periodicals, accompanied by a notation that all the books ordered from Europe had not yet arrived.

By 1807, when Warren assumed custody and shifted the Boston Medical Library a few blocks down Marlborough Street from Fleet's to Smith's, the European books apparently had made port; the catalogue listed 145 titles, with fifty-four more on order. . . in a fair way, at this rate, to crowd John Fleet out of his bachelor's haven after all. In 1808 the first official pharmacopoeia in the United States, compiled by Warren and Jackson, was published by the Massachusetts Medical Society, and the growing library was up to 223 titles. The one-share, one-book, borrowing regulation had been democratized to three titles at a time for one and all, and the trustees reserved the right to fine Apothecary Smith himself fifty cents a week for the heinous lapse of letting out a book and failing to record the fact. Their statement appended to this catalogue and dated May 30, 1808 is revealing:[10]

The Trustees of the Boston Medical Library have thought it might be agreeable to the Proprietors to receive, at the end of the third year, some general information of the state of the Library, and of such improvements as it is capable of receiving.

The Trustees cannot refrain from congratulating the Proprietors, that this establishment has progressed so rapidly, from a diminutive commencement, to its present importance and usefulness. Through its channels, the Physicians of this town are now constantly able to obtain the recent and valuable improvements made by the more advanced science of Europe. The library receives all the periodical publications of Great Britain, which relate to medical subjects. . . Nearly all other English Medical Publications, made since the formation of the library, have also been obtained. . . The most useful new works have been obtained from France. . . Besides these, the Trustees have paid for, and daily hope to receive from France, a most valuable Dictionary of Natural History, containing some hundreds of plates, a voluminous system of French Medical science, a condensed collection of the best French medical writers, and other new works. The medical publications of American Physicians have been procured without any exception, [not quite true. . . there was not a word by Benjamin Waterhouse, with whom Warren, Jackson and friends were on unfriendly terms]; of these are the New York Medical Repository, the Philadelphia Medical Museum—and Philadelphia Medical and Physical Journal, Rush's Medical Inquiries, Barton's Elements of Botany, &c. All these books are firmly and handsomely bound. The Trustees have lately ventured to add the 6 published volumes of Shaw's Zoology; a work, which can scarcely be rivalled in the beauty and accuracy of its representations of the various classes of the animal kingdom. . .

Whether this collection, placed in a convenient situation, accessible at all hours, has improved the state of medical knowledge among us, and increased the love of medical reading, the Trustees cannot undertake to say. They *can* say, that since the library has been opened, nearly seven hundred applications have been made for books, most of which would not have been seen in Boston, probably, had not this library existed [true enough. . . the catalogue listed "Catalogue Books of Boylston Library"]. . .

The Trustees are of opinion, and they think it their duty to suggest, that the library may be considerably and easily augmented. It must be confessed, that an accumulation of approved *old* works, would add much to its value, and form a

> solid foundation for this handsome structure. This might easily be effected by donations from the Proprietors, of some of the books in their libraries, which they have already perused. By this plan each would acquire the use of the combined contributions of his brethren. . . Should this take place, we might soon behold a collection of all the medical works, most important for study and for consultation; the acquisition of learning would be rendered easy, medical literature promoted, the present generation improved, and their successors inspired with emulation and gratitude.

The trustees acknowledged fifty donations of books, including twenty from Warren, thirteen from Jackson and ten from Coffin, and promised that the names of contributors would be "inscribed on a table [sic] suspended in the library." Their "handsome structure," however, was to remain at Smith's apothecary hardly longer than it had been in Dr. Fleet's charge. Personages and politics were pushing and pulling to move the whole body of the medical department under the Boston tent. In 1808 Warren's dissecting class at 49 Marlborough Street was augmented by the chemistry lectures of young Dr. John Gorham, a student of his father who had just married his sister, Mary Warren. Next year, on the recommendation of their respective faculty seniors, John Warren and Aaron Dexter, the two were elevated by the Harvard Corporation to adjunct professors of anatomy and surgery, and of chemistry and materia medica.

And then in midsummer of 1810 it all began to jell. The University approved the petition of the Warren-dominated medical faculty to open lectures in Boston. . . all save that eminent controversialist Benjamin Waterhouse, Hersey Professor of the Theory and Practise of Physic, the sole nonresident of Boston who was quite content to remain in Cambridge and continue lecturing a step or two from his door on Waterhouse Street. A few days later the Corporation came to an agreement with the overseers of the Leverett Street almshouse concerning the use of its clinical facilities for teaching, and at the same time created a new chair in clinical medicine to strengthen the Warrens' Boston cadre, appointing James Jackson its first occupant.

The squeeze was on Waterhouse, always happiest with his back to the wall. He protested with some justification that Jackson's chair was an encroachment on his own, but was overridden and forced by the Corporation to acquiesce formally to the extension of the School to Boston as the condition for his clinical privilege in the almshouse. In December of 1810 the six professors on Harvard's medical faculty (there were only eleven in the entire University) opened courses above White's apothecary in the rooms to which John Collins Warren had staked claim five years earlier. While cooperating ostensibly, Waterhouse after two months surfaced leading the unsuccessful effort of a claque of dissident physicians to gain incorporation from the General Court as the rival Massachusetts College of Physicians. Put down once again, the angry vaccinator lashed out libelously at his enemies; for this indiscretion he was discharged in 1812 from the Hersey professorship and suffered the wormwood of seeing it given to the mild James Jackson.

And so Harvard's medical department moved to Boston (all but abandoning its Boylston Medical Library),[11] and the Boston Medical Library, which by 1810 possessed 329 titles, moved (obedient to the Warren will) from 39 to 49 Marlborough Street to serve the needs of teacher and taught. When Thomas I. Parker was graduated in 1811, Dr. Warren turned the librarianship over to him. Little is remembered of Dr. Parker. He was born in Boston in 1784, took his degrees at Harvard and conveniently set up practice at 49 Marlborough where, Farlow states with interesting ambiguity, "he had charge of an electric machine and operated on patients from the Dispensary."[12]

While they were thus engaged, medical history records that Doctors Jackson and Warren also found the time in 1810 to issue a circular letter proposing the establishment of a teaching adjunct in Boston which the world would come to know as the Massachusetts General Hospital, and in 1812, with others of their circle, to publish the first number of a periodical outlet for the faculty, *The New England Journal of Medicine and Surgery.*

The success of their campaign to *extend*, as they euphemistically put it, Harvard's *medical establishment* to Boston and the luminescence of the pearl which another of their creations, the Boston Medical, or Second Social, Library had deposited around the catalytic collection of the Society for Medical Improvement, seem to have disposed the Improvers to let their Society quietly dissolve from the scene soon after 1810.[13] The Massachusetts Medical Society, inversely, flourished, while its library gathered cobwebs and was quite as quietly removed from its cloister in the home of John Fleet after his death in 1813, to reside once again alongside the robustious collection of the Medical Library at 49 Marlborough.

The Medical School throve in the fine, sickly environment of the growing, teeming, disease-ridden, accident-prone port of Boston, and the makeshift rooms over White's were, of course, ridiculously inadequate. Never ones to let the initiative slip, Warren, Jackson and the rest of the faculty persuaded the President and Fellows to request the General Court to finance a building of its own for the Medical School. Simultaneously they were pushing the trustees of the still nonexistent

Massachusetts General Hospital. In 1815 the Legislature voted funds for the construction of a medical school on Mason Street, opposite Boston Common, and gave the nascent hospital permission to enter the life insurance business, which it did after four years in the guise of the Massachusetts Hospital Life Insurance Company, and most profitably from that time forth.

"Taken altogether," wrote Boston chronicler Sam Drake of the new edifice of the Massachusetts Medical College (so named in gratitude to the legislators), "its external aspect might be called ugly."[14] Leaving 49 Marlborough to the pills and philters of the apothecaries, the delighted faculty and students moved into their brick schoolhouse in December 1816, just as the founders of the MGH opened a fund drive which resulted in five more years in the decidedly handsome granite structure designed by Charles Bulfinch. Were there borrowings, under Bulfinch's domed elegance, from the whimsical, balustraded, funnel-shaped affair that topped the Medical School's anatomical theatre, set so oddly upon an octagonal base which reared up with such squat complacence behind its excrescent pediment?

Provision had been made in the Mason Street horror for a library with a capacity of three thousand volumes, and when the medical faculty organized for the first time in November 1816 it voted to make a start by donating books which would be useful to the students. Dr. William Gamage, Jr., was appointed the librarian. He was the son of the doughty Cambridge allopathist, the memory of whom caused Dr. Holmes to shudder: "Grim, taciturn, rough in aspect, his visits to the household were the nightmare of the nursery."[15] The good intentions of the professors must have come to very little, for in 1819 the Boston Medical Library was again on the move, following the School with two thousand volumes, from Marlborough to Mason Street, to take its place beside Dr. Warren's swelling anatomical museum and to exert its gravitational pull on the lesser collections of the Massachusetts and Boylston medical societies which soon came to rest in the same queer structure that fifty years later, when it was serving humanity as a fire house, intrigued the inquisitive Drake to recall:

> Untold horrors were associated with this building in the minds of the urchins who frequented the adjoining schoolhouse. Its contiguity to the Common Burying-Ground, too, seemed to savor of a strong union between demand and supply. The professors were regarded in the neighborhood as so many ogres, and the students as no better than vampires. They ate their oysters or passed the jest over the dissecting-table with a *sang-froid* simply horrible to the uninitiated. An instance is remembered of a student, who went to pass the evening at a friend's house, taking a dead woman's arm, which he coolly unwrapped from a newspaper to the affright of his hostess.[16]

On May 3, 1826, after serving gratuitously for sixteen years as the Harvard Medical School's chief reference reliance, the Boston Medical Library was dissolved by its thirty-one proprietors, who ceded everything to the Boston Athenaeum in exchange for the privilege—which all but one picked up—of purchasing life subscriptions or proprietorships in that not yet venerable but already exceedingly private institution. James Jackson was no longer a proprietor of the Library, but John C. Warren, John Gorham and Jacob Bigelow were, and these four had been among the founders of the Anthology Society, later Club, gathered in 1804 to advance the literary amenities in Boston, which in 1807 adopted the evocative (and to the world beyond the pale, provocative) name, Athenaeum. The librarian who presided over this act of bibliothecarial self-immolation was Dr. George Hayward; a score of years hence, he and his old comrade-in-cutting Warren would perform civilization's first major surgery with ether anesthesia and add a name to the dome Bulfinch designed for the MGH.

The Boston Athenaeum in 1826 had occupied for only four years the mansion on Pearl Street, leading from Milk Street to the wharves, bequeathed it by James Perkins. The floors already were sagging under the weight of more than twenty thousand volumes when its full-blown medical department added more than another two thousand said to have been purchased within the decade at a cost to the Boston Medical Library of $4500, though regarded by their new owners as worth twice that.[17]

The rationale by which the proprietors, who comprised nearly half of the profession in the town, allowed their library after only twenty years of useful service to be absorbed by the Athenaeum has not survived. But a few inferences can be drawn. For one thing, every healthy independent library is an expanding organism, and the Medical Library's home, its host on Mason Street, was designed for three thousand volumes and no more.

The Athenaeum, for its part, had encountered financial problems the solution of which, in the studied opinion of its proprietors (a goodly share of them merchant princes), might lie in the assumption of an amoebic approach to its neighbors. To this end, the previous February they had appointed a committee under that resourceful mathematical genius from Salem, Nathaniel Bowditch, assigned to find ways and means "of uniting, in the Athenaeum, the principal circulating libraries of this city" with the object of filling the deficiencies in its collections. The prey must have been softened in advance, because on March 18 the

Athenaeum proprietors assembled in special meeting and blessed their projected union with the Boston Medical Library.

Other specialized libraries fell within the grasp of the Bowditch pseudopodium and added their substance to the cell on Pearl Street. The first to submit, even while the Medical Library was being digested, was the Massachusetts Scientific Library Association. Curiously, this society was only a few months old and possessed no books. Its owners, however, had already pledged $3700 toward the purchase of scientific volumes. Among them was John Collins Warren, a subscriber for fifty dollars.[18]

Evidently in the judgment of Dr. Warren the interests of the medical and scientific professions of the town at large—and of the three libraries he had taken a lead in creating—would best be served by their integration under one roof.

The twenty-nine of his thirty fellow proprietors of the Second Social, or first Boston Medical Library who reconvened with him in the parthenon on Park Street evidently agreed. The word of a Warren carried weight in the American Athens, generation unto generation.

2

Hibernation

1826 · 1874

Having struggled upriver to deposit the spawn from which sprang Boston's first medical library in 1805, the Society for Medical Improvement was wafted in a state of exhaustion back to the seas of oblivion. When it returned to life and to the stream in 1828, it was too late by two years to rescue its fingerling from the net of the Athenaeum. The Society was to swim in solitary self-improvement against the eddies of intellectual torpor which for another half a century, save for the appearance of a few productive upflows, would catch American medicine in their drift.

Boston had dozed along without an independent medical library for a generation when that first dermatologist, Dr. James C. White, opened practice in the middle of the century. Two score years later he looked back, unimpressed:

> It was truthfully said that the medical profession of Boston of those days lacked ambition. They were content to keep their knowledge to themselves, and to use it for their patients alone, or give expression to it through the restricted circles of these two small societies [Medical Improvement and Observation]. They rarely published a book, or lecture, or paper, and thus, with all the varied learning which some of them possessed in eminent degree, they held an inferior position to the physicians of other large cities of the country in the estimation of the medical world. I was for several years, 1863-1866, a co-editor of the *Boston Medical and Surgical Journal*, and remember the great difficulty it had in obtaining original articles from members of the profession here.[1]

Dr. White's junior, the widely published surgeon James G. Mumford, took the same occasion to wing a backward dart from the enlightened vantage of 1901 at Boston's first generation of medical Victorians. . . "those ancient men, our professional grandfathers, with their limited ideas of science as we know it; their strenuous gropings in the dark; their earnestness in small things; their blind pathology; their empirical therapeutics; their almost pathetic struggling toward the light."[2]

One who though strenuous did not grope, and who though struggling was not in the least pathetic, was Henry Ingersoll Bowditch, son of the great navigator who had charted the course which brought that first medical library and its cargo into the dry dock of the Athenaeum.

Dr. Bowditch was a handsome, broad-browed young man of twenty-three in 1832 when he was graduated from both Harvard Medical School and the Massachusetts General Hospital, where he was a house pupil under James Jackson, and sailed for France to join the pilgrimage from Boston and Philadelphia to Paris and the Aesculapian presence of Pierre Charles Alexandre Louis, who was shaking the medical world with his serene preachment of the revolutionary doctrine during his rounds of La Pitié that one should observe and think for himself. Oliver Wendell Holmes, who was Bowditch's junior by a year, joined him in Louis's clinic in the spring of 1833, and Henry wrote his father on May 12: "I had a talk a few days since with Holmes, who has been studying with Dr. Jackson, upon what I considered the advantages held out to a student in Paris, especially to a medical student when acquainted with Louis. We had a fight (as he called it) for an hour, and the next day I heard of his having said that either Louis was the greatest man that ever lived in medicine, or I was crazy."[3]

Another Parisian advantage that struck Bowditch was the accessibility of the libraries and museums to the public, so counter to Boston's private ways. "I will express my determination that upon my return," he promised his father in the same letter, "my grand aim shall be to give everybody the opportunity of study, and in this way repay to humanity at large the immense debt of gratitude I owe to France."

The first to whom Bowditch communicated his enthusiasm for Louis on his arrival home was John Ware, Adjunct Hersey Professor of the Theory and Practice of Physic.[4] A few months later, in 1835, the two organized the Boston Society for Medical Observation, with four medical students. It was a copy, even to the name, of Louis's Paris club, and its object was the same: to cultivate the habits of accurate clinical observation and case recording. Student interest proved ephemeral. In 1838 the Observation Society lapsed into dormancy. But in March 1846, that year of American decision, Bowditch breathed into it life anew, possibly inspired by the vote of the faculty some weeks earlier urging that a new medical school be erected on a lot of flats on North Grove Street given by Dr. George Parkman, a few steps from the MGH. For their part, the trustees of the Hospital countervoted "that they cannot perceive any advantage to this institution to arise therefrom."[5]

What did arise from their deliberations were, first, the east wing of the Bulfinch Building in July of 1846, then a year hence, the west, which together doubled its capacity and bracketed in place and time Gilbert

Abbott's ethereal triumph over pain while stretched out in the surgical amphitheatre in between on October 16, 1846. Bowditch and Holmes were appointed visiting physicians early that year. Harvard's Massachusetts Medical College leapfrogged Beacon Hill from Mason to North Grove Street at the end of 1847, a little beyond an end of the Hospital's decrepit wooden fence, regarding which a neighbor with plaintive futility once remarked to trustee N. I. Bowditch, "Your institution always reminds me of a fine, likely-looking man disfigured by a rusty coat and a 'shocking bad hat.' "[6]

The move gave rise to a larger faculty and somewhat of a new order at the School. Holmes was made the first Parkman Professor of Anatomy and Physiology in honor of that ill-starred donor of the mud flat on which its foundation floated, and his fellow professors elected him their dean to succeed Dr. Walter Channing. Forty-four years afterward the aged anatomist dissected in friendly fashion his associates of '47 in a letter to Dr. James Read Chadwick, the founding librarian of the Medical Library of which Holmes was the first president. This hitherto unpublished communication was a salute to the first annual meeting of the Harvard Medical Alumni Association, which Chadwick also founded. Dr. Holmes was eighty-one and in his North Shore cottage for the summer.[7]

Beverly Farms, Mass.
June 19, 1891.

Dear Dr. Chadwick,

I regret that I shall not be able to attend the meeting of the Medical School Association on the 23rd of this month.

I send my heartiest greetings to the Association. I know the members would receive me kindly as a relic of the past not without a certain value as a fragment of antiquity. I have long been the sole survivor of that primeval Faculty of which I became a member in 1847. In that point of view I am not merely a rarity, I am a unique specimen, and have an adventitious market price like one of those rare cents for which collectors pay a premium. Half worn out old copper as it is, its scarcity makes it worth a dime or perhaps a dollar.

In the days to which I refer the Faculty could say of itself in the words of Wordsworth's little girl

"We are seven"

John Ware, cautious, conscientious, thoughtful, quiet, judicious; Jacob Bigelow, sagacious, independent, with grave aspect, and an inner consciousness full of fun and satire, a man of many accomplishments, but above all of soundness and practical wisdom; Walter Channing, sanguine, enthusiastic, hospitable to new ideas of all sorts, with something of the literary tastes and tendencies belonging to the family of which he was a member; George Hayward, eminently social and a very agreeable companion, old-fashioned in various ways—he always made a pīnt of saying jīnt for joint—eminent as a surgeon, but rather too nervous for a model operator. Of the three others one name must be passed over in silence—it is too well remembered without being spoken. The two others of the seven were

Dr. John Barnard Swett Jackson and myself, who became members of the Faculty in that same year, 1847.

Of Dr. John Jackson it is impossible to speak without an affectionate tribute—to his pure, transparent, truthful nature, joined with a love for the most unlovely department of anthropology, the study of diseased and degenerated human organs—a love like that of an artist for his more alluring pursuit. The monuments of his industry are to be seen and studied in our museums. So long as he lived the citizen of Boston could say truly, if there was anything interesting in his fatal illness, *non omnis moriar*, for some portion of his bodily frame was sure to be saved from decay and skillfully prepared and arranged by our expert colleague to survive in alcoholic immortality.

Two years after I became a member of the Faculty the name of Henry Jacob Bigelow was added to the list of its members. His eulogy has so lately been spoken that I will not repeat the language with which his ablest contemporaries have done honor to his memory, nor say over what I myself have placed upon the record elsewhere. I will only add here that strenuous as he was in any labor which interested, he was most vivacious and entertaining in the interests of business—playful, often, as the young kitten of a lioness.

During a large part of my period of service as Professor, I enjoyed the companionship of Dr. David Humphreys Storer, the only other survivor besides myself of the ancient, primeval Faculty. Ardent, impulsive, indefatigable in the branch of the profession to which he especially devoted himself, Dr. Storer was preeminently the friend of the medical student. There was nothing he would not do to serve a pupil, and I trust that he will be remembered by the Alumni of the School at this, their first meeting, in accents which will reach him in his chamber of age and infirmity.

I have grown prolix with my recollections and I will close at once by wishing long life and all prosperity to the Association of the Alumni of the Medical School of Harvard University.

Very truly yours,
O. W. Holmes[8]

Possibly emboldened by his elevation with Holmes to a physicianship at the MGH, and the presumed availability of space within the new wings, (or the ten-year tenure on the board of his elder brother Nathaniel), Henry Ingersoll Bowditch communicated to the trustees on November 21, 1847 his concern over their failure to implement a medical library at the Hospital in spite of their assignment of a two-member committee in 1844 to spend fifty dollars for the purpose. The trustees were preoccupied with the tragic controversy which was clouding the ether euphoria, but they obliged with another $250 and allowed that "an annual appropriation will probably be continued for this object." In 1848 they appointed him the Hospital's first librarian, with 103 volumes in his care, and he had a bookplate designed and engraved.[9]

The poverty of medical literature in Boston weighed on Dr. Bowditch. He got behind a move in the Observation Society to subscribe to nine journals for circulation to members. In 1849 he was recording secretary of a select committee of the Massachusetts Medical Society to investigate its own neglected library which had been shuffled about in one after another dust-bestirring move from the Mason Street medical school to the Society's quarters behind the Athenaeum on Pearl Street, thence to its most recent place of repose in the Masonic Temple at Tremont Street and Temple Place. An inventory revealed that 280 of the 744 volumes were missing. The Fellows were enjoined to turn in their truants, and locks were put on the bookcases.

It was at this time that Bowditch made his most significant contribution to clinical medicine, his paper "On Pleuritic Effusions, and the Necessity of Paracentesis for Their Removal" which he read before the Observation Society on October 20, 1851. This observation *par excellence* was the product of his long interest in the chest and of his collaboration with Dr. Morrill Wyman of Cambridge, who had demonstrated the effectiveness of tapping with trocar and suction pump.

Bowditch was a restless soul, inquisitive, interested in everything and everyone, socially very conscious, deeply distressed by the state of the Union, a man of extraordinary benevolence. Had he concentrated his energies on Boston's medical bibliographic problem in the fulness of his career, he might have revived an independent library, but it is doubtful. At mid-century, the pressures were not great; not until the germ theory broke on the world, was the literature let loose.

Nor was Harvard in the vanguard of medical learning, or indeed, education. Years before, Ward Nicholas Boylston's hopeful legacy had gone awry with the move of Harvard's medical department to Boston. In 1851 it was uselessly stashed in the interior of the college library, some thousand volumes, as Harvard Librarian Thaddeus W. Harris reported on December 9, "mostly of the ancient standard authors. I am not aware that any additions have been made to it for twenty years or more." There were also at Cambridge as many medical works again, thought Harris, of which a number were duplicates of the Boylston collection, "but very few published within the present century."[10] The lot was available to medical faculty and students with the time and inclination to cross the river on an expedition into antiquity, and even to Fellows of the Massachusetts Medical Society if they lived within ten miles of the Yard.

In frustration, Dr. Horatio R. Storer, son of David Humphreys Storer and secretary of the Boylston Medical Society, begged the Harvard Corporation on January 3, 1852 to release the Boylston Library to the School, or at least the books in the college library which were not restricted by deed of gift, for the works in Cambridge were simply not accessible to the Boston students. . . "unconsulted and unconsultable." The Medical School library contained only 1200 books, Dr. Storer complained.[11] But apparently to no avail.

In an odd quirk of events, it was a literary Lafayette from France who turned the tide for public enlightenment and assisted Bostonians in loosening the monopoly of the private libraries. Nicholas Marie Alexandre Vattemare was an unlikely hero, a former stage ventriloquist who had abandoned the boards, possessed by *une grande fantaisie* of a world united in cultural brotherhood through an international exchange of books. M. Vattemare created great popular excitement when he burst upon Boston in 1841 with his proposition to weld together all of the local private libraries into a single great public one. But bellwethers such as the Athenaeum and the Society for Medical Improvement broke the chain by declining to be links. Vattemare was undiscouraged. In a *tour de force* of his specialty, he departed Boston but left his presence behind, and for an encore projected several gifts of books clear across from Paris. These feats stimulated those who had fallen within his spell to organize the Boston Public Library in 1852. It opened in Mason Street in two more years. It was better than no repository at all for the private collections of physicians no longer wanted by themselves, and certainly not by their heirs.[12]

For the practitioner the opening of the Boston Public Library, with the natural reluctance of its librarian to invest in a highly technical collection, was not the answer. Geographically it was as much a hindrance as bibliographically it was a help. Dr. David Williams Cheever recalled the beginnings of his surgical practice after his graduation from Harvard Medical School in 1858:

> I remember myself, when trying to look up subjects, vibrating between the Boston Athenaeum, which had some medical books, and the Public Library, which had other medical books, and the library in Temple Place, which belonged to the Improvement Society; so that the scanty sources of knowledge that existed then were scattered in three places, and great waste of time and patience was the result.[13]

Dr. Cheever's only clinical alliance would be with the Boston City Hospital when it opened in 1864, so his bookhunting vibrations would not customarily have penetrated the MGH's shocking bad fence into its staff library. This sanctum, after getting off to its shaky start under the prodding of Dr. Bowditch, was the beneficiary of a most eccentrically arranged bequest in 1858, the excellent medical library of the late Dr. John G. Treadwell of Salem, enriched with a noble endowment of $5000. Treadwell's gift redounded to the Hospital after rebounding off the President and Fellows of Harvard College, who rejected it earlier in the year owing to what they considered the "unusual and embarrassing conditions" he had attached to his first intention that his alma mater should be his beneficiary. The doctor died in 1856. He drew his strange will in 1847, the year of Henry Bowditch's first concern with the MGH library. Both were Salem natives; Treadwell graduated from the Medical School in 1828, four years ahead of Bowditch.

The conditions which caused such embarrassment would have required the University to create a chair for a "Teacher of Physiology," to be endowed by Treadwell according to pages upon pages of the most impossible restrictions and instructions as to the holder's qualifications, selection and duties, and to maintain the Treadwell collection intact, adding to it only from unexpended income. Should Harvard decline or fail to comply with any of the preposterous conditions, everything was to go to the Hospital. . . and under the most rational and straightforward circumstances, hardly a string attached. Evidently Dr. Treadwell had taken a scunner at the Medical School. His will is an extraordinary aberration.[14]

Charles W. Eliot's famous rejoinder of 1870 to Dr. Henry Jacob Bigelow's sarcastic wonderment why reforms should be proposed in *his* medical school. . . "There is a new President". . . marks as well as any five words can the rush of events which overtook American medicine in that postwar decade. There was a new President of Harvard, and a new science.

Mr. Eliot nailed his thesis to the door on North Grove Street in his first annual report of January 1871: "The whole system of medical education in this country needs thorough reformation. The course of professional instruction should be a progressive one covering three years; the Winter Session and the Summer Session should be combined; and the student should give his attendance at lectures and recitations, at hospitals and laboratories during the whole year." From his own experience lecturing in chemistry at the School, Eliot was appalled at the absence of dialogue between teacher and students, many of whom he found to be semiliterate. He thought it a miracle that Harvard produced any good doctors at all.[15]

As for the new science, Dr. J. Collins Warren, son of Dr. Jonathan Mason Warren, grandson of Dr. John Collins Warren, Great-Grandson of Dr. John Warren, brought a souvenir of it back to Boston from Europe. It was a small supply of Joseph Lister's dressings and an inexhaustible one of fervor for antisepsis, which this beginner of twenty-seven employed in an unheard-of fashion for the first time during a mastectomy on October 9, 1869. Dr. Bigelow had already rejected carbolic acid, as he had Eliot, but in time he came to accept both, as Margaret Fuller in her time did the universe.

The biological sciences were about to fruit wildly in the medium mixed by Pasteur. But how well prepared for it was America? How well stocked in Boston was the larder of the laboratory, the library? Truly Diogenic now in the length and breadth of beard and wisdom, Henry Ingersoll Bowditch kept aloft his light, and lamented the leanness of the literature. Membership in the Medical Observation Society had taken a rise after Dr. Bowditch introduced the "clinical conference" (borrowed from the admired Louis) when he came into the Jackson professorship of clinical medicine in 1859. By 1871 the whole picture was changing, and periodicals were coming into such demand that the Society found it necessary to divide itself into four classes, of which only the honorary and active (limited to forty) retained the privilege to borrow from the twenty-five journals now subcribed to.

Desiccate as the dust that drifted down upon it, the library of the Massachusetts Medical Society drowsed on. The librarian reported dryly in 1864 that "one member of the Society had, during the year, intimated an intention of taking out books, but had not done so." This negative statistic distressed the Fellows, and they appointed a new librarian, Dr. James C. White. Five years passed, and he had to confess that during all of 1870 no one had so much as intimated that he might consult the collection. He recommended that it be dispersed, Fellows to get first crack, the rest to be deposited in a public library. The Council so voted in June 1872, and the Society's entire stock, consisting of 1687 uncracked books, 9201 unconsulted pamphlets and sixteen unappreciated broadsides, was sent over to the Boston Public Library.

This was too much for Dr. Bowditch. He was a former trustee of the Public Library and as loyal to it as anyone, but the mass of material which the Society had let go included all of its archives, much of which he had painstakingly collected in three folio volumes, the Bowditch Books, when he was secretary between 1849 and 1854. He protested, but too late; the Council confirmed the transfer on June 4, 1874.[16]

By 1874 President Eliot had so far succeeded in reshaping the Harvard Medical School into his image of the future of medical education, and in bringing around the Old Guard, that on October 22 the faculty was right behind him at a spirited meeting to kick off a $200,000 campaign for a new building. Governor J. H. Clifford and Eliot shared the rostrum with Edward Everett Hale, who declared sonorously that he was ashamed of Boston's meagre support of medical education. . . "we cannot afford to play second fiddle to Paris or London." Of course the day belonged to Dr. Holmes. With feeling he dwelt on the inflammability of the North Grove Street fire trap and expressed his conviction that the Warren Anatomical Museum and the library deserved ample halls and endowment. . .

I carried a gentleman recently graduated at Dublin University only yesterday to the medical college, and was made to feel this first want most keenly. The one preparation which I most wished to show him was not in the museum, where it was not thought safe to keep it, on account of the risk of fire, but deposited in the building of the Society of Natural History. I did not ask him to look at the library, which is not what it should be; does not grow as it should, and never will until it is removed from an inflammable building and a most dangerous neighborhood.[17]

The Governor appointed a Committee of Fifty lay and medical men to go after the money. The penultimate name belonged to Dr. James Read Chadwick, a youthful instructor in gynecology who had lately been let in to the Observation Society, which was to a man almost one with the faculty.[18] Chadwick was ten days short of thirty, an ebullient, Bohemian sort of fellow, rather romantic in his tastes, a fancy and striking dresser, with just that bit of airiness and flair about him which seems to be a requisite for the specialty he chose. He was a Boston boy, came along the Harvard way, and the year he graduated from the Medical School, in 1871, married Katherine Lyman, daughter of Dr. George H. Lyman, a handsome aristocrat of "democratic" manner who had served as one of the six medical inspectors in the Union Army during the Civil War. After his mustering-out Dr. Lyman took up gynecology, which could explain his son-in-law's choice of specialty if not of wife. Too, Chadwick was an ardent admirer of his old anatomy professor whose great contribution to obstetrics and gynecology on "The Contagiousness of Puerperal Fever" of thirty-one years past was well known to him; nor was he deaf at this gala fundraising event for which Dr. Holmes was the star attraction to those sardonic cracks about the Medical School's impoverished library, too shameful to be shown to the visitor from Ireland.

Chadwick certainly was aware at this time of the really embarrassing state that the profession in Boston had allowed its reference literature to fall into, most acutely so as he entered practice and teaching after his postgraduate tour of the European centers with his bride the previous summer of 1873. It appears to have been in 1874 that he took his first interest in the proposition that Boston ought to have a decent medical library. He put out some feelers to a few of the leaders in the profession and got negative response, and he didn't do much better with Justin Winsor, Librarian of the Boston Public Library, who only let him have some duplicates of the antique Medical Society collection.

It is not impossible to imagine that Dr. Chadwick's enthusiasm for a medical library was as fortuitous as the manner of his stumbling upon a career, as related by his successor in the enterprise, Dr. Farlow:

While in Vienna in June, 1867, dining at the Riedhof with some of his medical American friends, he [Chadwick] deplored his aimless and useless life and asked whether anyone could tell him what line of work he could take up with any prospect of success. One of the number replied, "Jim, study medicine; you would make a good doctor." This suggestion was greeted with explosive laughter as being too absurd for serious consideration. This seemingly ridiculous advice apparently appealed to him, he returned to Boston and entered the Harvard Medical School the following autumn.[19]

Perhaps during an evening's joust with kindred spirits of the Medical Observation Society, where the influence of Henry Ingersoll Bowditch was felt above all others, talk turned to the damned inexcusable unavailability of the medical literature in town and someone challenged: "Jim, why don't you get up a decent library? You're just the man to do it."

And so he did. On December 21, 1874, two months almost to the day after Dr. Holmes had confessed his chagrin on that score, six Observation members assembled in Dr. Bowditch's office at 113 Boylston Street to organize a medical library. The catalyst, young Chadwick, was chosen secretary and wrote up the minutes:

On Tuesday, December 21, 1874, six gentlemen, Drs. H. I. Bowditch, S. A. Green, R. T. Edes, Thomas Dwight, F. I. Knight, and J. R. Chadwick, met at the office of Dr. Bowditch, 113 Boylston St., for the purpose of taking measures to secure the speedy establishment of a Medical Library in the City of Boston. The meeting was organized by the election of Dr. Green as Chairman and Dr. Chadwick as Secretary. Those who had called the meeting then pointed out the urgent need of such an institution, referred to the magnificent collections of books in other cities and expressed the opinion that we ought to have, and could have, a Medical Library in Boston if proper steps were taken to obtain it.

The efforts that had been made for two or three years past in the Observation Society, looking to the establishment of a library and reading room in connection with that Society, were alluded to, and a conviction expressed by several of those present that a separate Association, whose sole aim and object should be the collection and preservation of books, would insure our having the best Library in the end.

After a very brief discussion these views were acquiesced in by all the gentlemen present; but, as the comparative advantages of one plan or the other could not, and ought not to be determined without due reflection, as the cooperation and contributions of the various societies, notably of the Observation Society, were essential to the success of the project, it was unanimously voted to postpone all action until the sentiments of the Societies had been sounded.

Dr. Dwight and the Secretary were then appointed a committee to confer with the officers and members of the Medical Societies and secure, if possible, their sanction and assistance.

Adjourned to Tuesday, December 28, 1874.

JAMES R. CHADWICK, M.D.[20]

All were Harvard Medical School graduates. Bowditch was their Nestor, chairman now of the Massachusetts Board of Health, second such in the country. Samuel Abbott Green was forty-four, a bachelor, bibliophile, antiquarian and politician. . . that is, City Physician, trustee of the Boston Public Library, and future mayor. Robert T. Edes, from Eastport, Maine, was thirty-six, a scholar, Assistant Professor of Materia Medica and concerned with diseases of the nervous system, which would lead him to running the Adams Nervine Asylum and some early work in the treatment of psychoneuroses. Frederick I. Knight had trained with Dr. Austin Flint in New York and Bowditch in Boston, hence his interest in laryngology; he was thirty-three and Instructor in Auscultation, Percussion and Laryngoscopy. Thomas Dwight was thirty-one, Instructor in Comparative Anatomy and Histology at Harvard, Professor of Anatomy at Bowdoin College Medical School and editor of the *Boston Medical and Surgical Journal*; in nine years he would have the awesome job of filling the Parkman chair vacated by Holmes. The youngest, Chadwick, was just thirty.

It was perfectly appropriate that after forty-eight years of interment the soul of the first Boston Medical Library should have been released in the office of Henry Ingersoll Bowditch. Thus was consummated his love of medicine and learning, and the pledge of an idealistic young medical student under the spell of a great clinician, sworn to an honored father, that *my grand aim shall be to give everybody the opportunity of study, and in this way to repay to humanity at large the immense debt of gratitude I owe to France.*

3

The Pied Piper of Hamilton Place

1875 · 1877

Christmas came and went (not so merrily to a nation still paying for the panic of '73), and on December 28, 1874 the six medical gentlemen proposing to fill the library void in Boston reconvened. They had bent the holiday to their purpose, and now they were nineteen, all but one members of the Medical Observation Society. As before, Samuel Abbott Green presided. The merits of a mere expansion of the Society's periodical collection against the creation of an independent library of books and journals around this nucleus were debated. The majority favored transplanting to new ground, but a few hesitated to deflower the old club, and the issue was unresolved.[1]

Youth, or the youthful outlook, zeal in the new science, and Harvard Medical School were the touchstones of the nineteen. All were alumni, fourteen within ten years, thirteen in the classes between '65 and '69. Fourteen were faculty. Henry Ingersoll Bowditch, the inspirer of it all, was the revered graybeard; he had relinquished the Jackson professorship in 1867. Senior active faculty was Francis Minot (HMS 1844), Hersey Professor of the Theory and Practice of Medicine (Medicine now, not Physic) since the previous May. He was with Chadwick, Bowditch, Edes, Knight and Bowditch's nephew, Henry Pickering Bowditch (1868), strong for a separate library. H. P. was Assistant Professor of Physiology; he set up the first physiological laboratory in America in the attic of the North Grove Street school and was well on his brilliant way. So was his classmate, Reginald Heber Fitz, Assistant Professor of Pathological Anatomy; from Rudolf Virchow's lab in Berlin, Fitz had just carried cellular pathology to America.

Inclined protectively toward their Observation Society collection with Fitz were Edward Wigglesworth (1865), Instructor in Dermatology; William Lambert Richardson (1867), the Instructor in Obstetrics who a year earlier had singlehandedly spanked the Boston Lying-In Hospital back to life after sixteen comatose years; and J. Collins (Coll) Warren (1866), Instructor in Surgery. Productive minds.

Of the remaining seven, Clarence J. Blake (1865) was the School's first Lecturer in Otology, one rung ahead of John O. Green (1866), instructor in this new specialty. Charles Pickering Putnam (1869), a grandson of James Jackson, was Lecturer on the Diseases of Children. Blake and Putnam would be heard from; they were in Chadwick's camp. Putnam's classmate, Frank W. Draper, was Lecturer on Hygiene and interesting himself in legal medicine, which would lead to his appointment as the first Suffolk County medical examiner, first in Massachusetts. Charles E. Stedman (1855) was in general practice and obstetrics, visiting at Boston City Hospital. Arthur H. Nichols (1866) was a GP, and so was Edward J. Forster (1868), an obstetrician-gynecologist in Charlestown and the only one of the nineteen not recorded on the Observation roster.[2]

Through the winter and into the summer of 1875 the meetings continued, and Chadwick the proselytizer prevailed. The doubters were converted, the misgivings of older members were overridden, and the Observation Society voted to deposit its journals with the proposed Medical Library Association. On the first of August, Knight, Wigglesworth, Richardson and Chadwick sent around a circular[3] summoning an organizational meeting for the twentieth in the rooms of the Massachusetts Medical Society at 36 Temple Place. It began:

> *Whereas*, The need has long been felt among the members of the Medical Profession in this vicinity, of an opportunity to consult, at will, the Standard Medical Works and the files of the current Medical Periodicals, it has been thought that the size of the Profession is now such as to warrant the formation of a Medical Library Association, to meet the above want.
>
> Several large collections of books have already been placed at our disposal, and many periodicals, now taken by clubs and individuals, will be transferred to this Association for binding and preservation. As the Library is intended especially for reference, it will not be allowable to take any books except duplicates from the rooms. It is proposed to keep the rooms open throughout the day and evening, during which time a competent person will be in attendance. . .

It was stated that two rooms in a house in Hamilton Place, a retired nook off Tremont Street across from the Park Street Church, were "most admirably adapted to the purposes of the Library" on good terms. The annual assessment was proposed to be ten dollars.

A hundred favorable replies were received, and twenty-three assembled at Temple Place on August 20, 1875, including only half of the December nineteen, probably due to the out-of-town attractions of summer vacation. Everything had been organized with Chadwickian efficiency. Knight called the meeting to order. Richardson and C. E. Inches were nominated chairman and secretary pro tem. The purpose of the gathering was explained. On motion of Chadwick, the chair appointed him, Blake and Moses W. Weld to compose a constitution and by-laws. They retired for a few moments and returned with the document as if handed to them on the mountain top. After some amendment it was adopted. It set forth that the objects of the Boston Medical Library Association were "to form a Library of medical and scientific books, journals and pamphlets for ready reference; to render the current medical periodicals at once accessible to the profession generally, and to establish a place of resort for the medical profession." Admission was to be open to members of the Massachusetts Medical and Dental societies, the Massachusetts College of Pharmacy and such others as might be anointed by the committee on admission. There would be an executive committee of which the unpaid Librarian was to be chairman ex officio, and a paid assistant librarian to have charge of everything, under his direction. Annual dues, ten dollars.

Fitz then moved the appointment of a nominating committee. No sooner said than done, and in a twinkling he, R. L. Hodgdon and John H. McCollum submitted a full slate of officers headed by Oliver Wendell Holmes, which was promptly elected. The meeting adjourned, and the Boston Medical Library Association was alive and breathing, lacking only a lease and a functioning subaltern for its founding Librarian, James Read Chadwick.

By what persistent persuasion, by what endearing processes of erosion, Chadwick captured the elderly and eminent anatomist and man of letters, now upon the heights of his fame, to lead off the letterhead of his library can be deduced from this wry tip of the Holmesian pen to

> the men who first met together, the men who have given their time and money, the faithful workers, worthy associates of the strenuous agitator who gave no sleep to his eyes, no slumber to his eyelids, until he had gained his ends; the untiring, imperturbable, tenacious, irrepressible, all-subduing agitator who neither rested nor let others rest until the success of the project was assured. If, against his injunctions, I name Dr. James Read Chadwick, it is only my revenge for his having kept me awake so often and so long while he was urging on the undertaking in which he had been preeminently active and triumphantly successful.[4]

Dr. Holmes's vice president was quite the opposite of him in temper. Dr. Charles E. Buckingham was fifty-five, Harvard Medical School 1844, where he was Professor of Obstetrics and Medical Jurisprudence. He was Henry Bowditch's strong ally in pushing for the first state board of health, of like stripe with Bowditch and Chadwick in their espousal of the right of women to medical education. "In his early professional career," Harrington wrote of him, "Buckingham was often in sore straits; his means were small, and he was without family influence and social connection. . . The struggle. . . left its scars, and one finds him afterwards a bitter and sometimes a censorious critic of men possessing those advantages which he had lacked. No one, however, was more just than he in giving praise to those whom he thought had honestly won position. Few men of his time wielded a more trenchant pen, or were more ready to debate than he."[5]

One who *was* well matched in council with Dr. Buckingham was the first secretary and ex officio chairman of the committee on admission, Oliver Fairfield Wadsworth (HMS 1865), of exact mentality and habit, an ophthalmologist and intimate of Fitz, H. P. Bowditch, the psychologist William James and others of a small and vigorous circle with whom he fled on vacations to an Adirondacks cabin summer after summer. Wadsworth loved the outdoors, athletics, music, literature, the company of friends, and not least, strong argument and disputation, for the warmth of it no less than the light. "It was a marked characteristic of him," wrote one of them, "that he could differ from his friends most fundamentally yet without any breach of friendship. He said exactly what he thought, and maintained his opinions vigorously, but there was never bitterness in his arguments. On the contrary, a twinkle of the eye, a winning smile and a merry word were always ready."[6]

Amos L. Mason was the first treasurer. He came up from Salem, specializing in contagious diseases. Dr. Mason was a year behind Chadwick at the Medical School and lived almost directly across Clarendon Street from him, within easy reach of the long arm.

On the first of October Chadwick hired Dr. Edwin Howard Brigham as his Assistant Librarian at twenty-five dollars a month. Like Chadwick, Brigham had backed into medicine. He was twenty-one at the outbreak of the Civil War, with no career prospects, and joined up as a private in the Thirteenth Massachusetts Volunteer Infantry. He was captured in the Second Battle of Bull Run on August 30, 1862, only to be turned loose by the Rebs in the countryside in a few weeks, sick with the runs, to make his way north. "While passing through Hagerstown, Maryland, [he] dropped from exhaustion in front of the house of a kindly old German, a grape grower, who took him in, nursed him and gave him money with which to reach home as soon as he was able to move. The friendship thus loyally and romantically begun was kept up until the death of the good Samaritan, and Dr. Brigham made several visits to Hagerstown to see him after the war was over."[7]

Convalescing in Boston, Private Brigham was befriended by a hard-drinking Army surgeon, A. N. McLaren, who helped him qualify as a hospital steward in 1864 and urged him to apply, successfully, for admission to Harvard Medical School, from which he graduated in 1868.[8] Surgeon Brigham remained in the Army in Boston, examining recruits among other duties, and crossed paths with Dr. Henry I. Bowditch, who had concerned himself with the problems of the veterans, as with everything else. In February of 1875 Brigham assisted Bowditch in preparing a paper which his patron presented before the Thursday Evening Club. Here Brigham met Chadwick, with whose father-in-law, George H. Lyman, he had been acquainted from war days when Lyman was an Army medical inspector.

Disinclined toward practice on account of his health and temperament, Brigham resigned from the Army for a job as clerk for the State Board of Health, of which Bowditch was chairman. That August the Medical Library was reborn. Chadwick and Bowditch (not to mention H. P. Bowditch, an HMS classmate of Brigham) induced him to take responsibility for the rooms now hired at 5 Hamilton Place in the mornings, while handling the duties of his Board of Health clerkship there during afternoons. By this arrangement he had a small living. After the Library's hours settled down to nine to six, Custodian-Clerk Brigham had to wear two hats between lunch and dinner. He was an affable factotum, the ideal *fides Achates* for the restless Chadwick, placid in the pleasant pace of his modest sinecure.

The two rooms of the Boston Medical Library Association opened for members on Monday, October 18, 1875.

> Each room was about eighteen feet square and had a door opening from the corridor leading from the street. The front room had one large window and a door with a large glass, which was always kept closed, where Dr. Brigham sat at a writing table formerly belonging to Dr. James Jackson. In the center was a large round table. . . There were also a large easy-chair and twelve black walnut cane-seated chairs. . . On shelves in a small alcove were kept the subscription journals. The rear room had rows of shelves about the walls and in the centre with a capacity of twenty-five hundred or more volumes. This room had large windows looking out on to a deep yard, so that there was plenty of light. Overhead were the quiet rooms of the Episcopal Church Association.
>
> Hamilton Place was then a very peaceful spot and near the business section. There was no entrance to Music Hall from it at that time. On both sides were old, well-built dwelling houses in a stage of transition to business purposes. It was closed at the end, and people from out of town used to hitch their horses here while on shopping bent.[9]

Boston's 648 square feet of medical library, including toilet, created no great stir at first. The times were hard, the doubters in the profession dismissed it as foolhardy, and the heft of the senior men thought it redundant to their main reliance, the *Boston Medical and Surgical Journal* and *Braithwaite,* an abstract of English periodicals. Not, in fact, until the *Index Medicus* and *Index Catalogue* began to issue forth from the Surgeon General's Library in 1879 and 1880, reforming the undisciplined horde of medical literature into a magnificent and well-ordered legion, did Chadwick have a matrix of ranks and files to fill with all the passion of his rage for recruitment. It is delightful to discover the man responsible for the conception and execution of the truly grand strategy of the *Indices*, Dr. John Shaw Billings, writing to Chadwick a week to the day after the opening of the new Library in Boston:

War Department,
Surgeon General's Office,
Washington, D.C., Oct. 25th 1875.

Dear Doctor,

I am at my desk again, physically weary, but mentally refreshed.

I am sitting in the midst of heaps of books, and with a table which is the personification of Chaos. All of which suits me exactly. I have sent you by express a package of books for the library of your new Society, and when you come on I shall have something for yourself personally. Please present my best respects to Mrs. Chadwick, and tell her that her selections have great and unmixed satisfaction.

Mrs Billings sends her love to Mrs C——.

"Mammy Helen" has worn a broad grin ever since my return.

My three days with you are marked in my memory with the largest white Stone I have ever set up.

I write in haste, as I have a large sheaf of letters to answer.

Very sincerely your friend
J S Billings[10]

The writer was a tall, commanding personality of thirty-seven who concealed a quirk of whimsy and fun behind the hedge, nay, the bush, of his formidable mustache, a Herculean worker, impatient with pretension in any form, a scorner of fools and a genius at creative organization. After completing the course at the Medical College of Ohio he entered the Army and rose during the Civil War to be one of the six medical inspectors, with Chadwick's father-in-law, George Lyman; possibly it was through Lyman that the two medical librarians met. In 1865 Billings was assigned to the Surgeon General's office and given charge of its library of about 2200 volumes. By 1871 he had beefed this up to 13,330 with an $80,000 "slush fund" turned back by Army hospitals after the war and moved the library into the Army Medical Museum, which had taken over the infamous Ford's, now no longer a theatre. Thus, out of an Ohio medical student's frustration with the jungle of the literature while trying to research his thesis was conceived the National Library of Medicine.

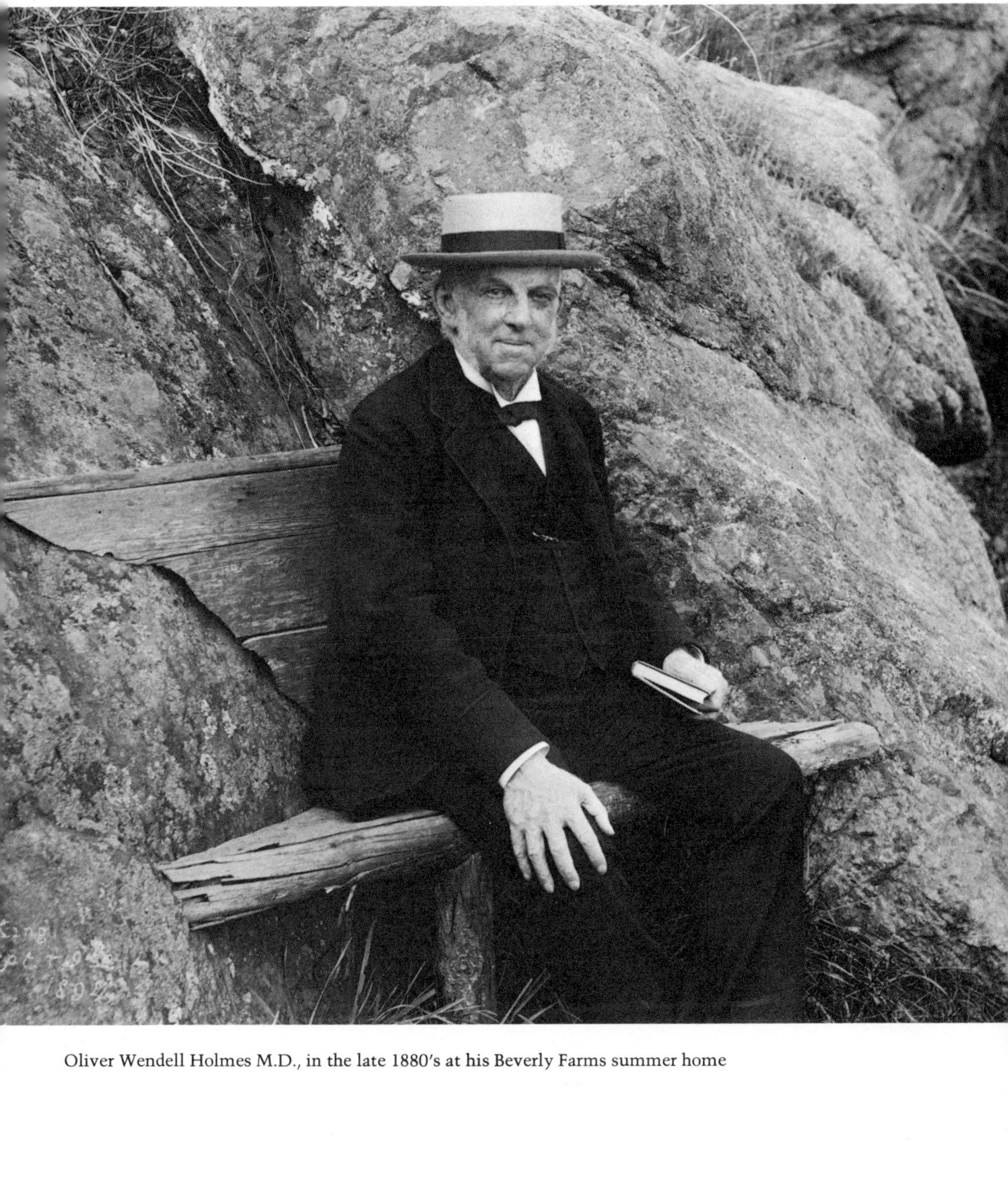

Oliver Wendell Holmes M.D., in the late 1880's at his Beverly Farms summer home

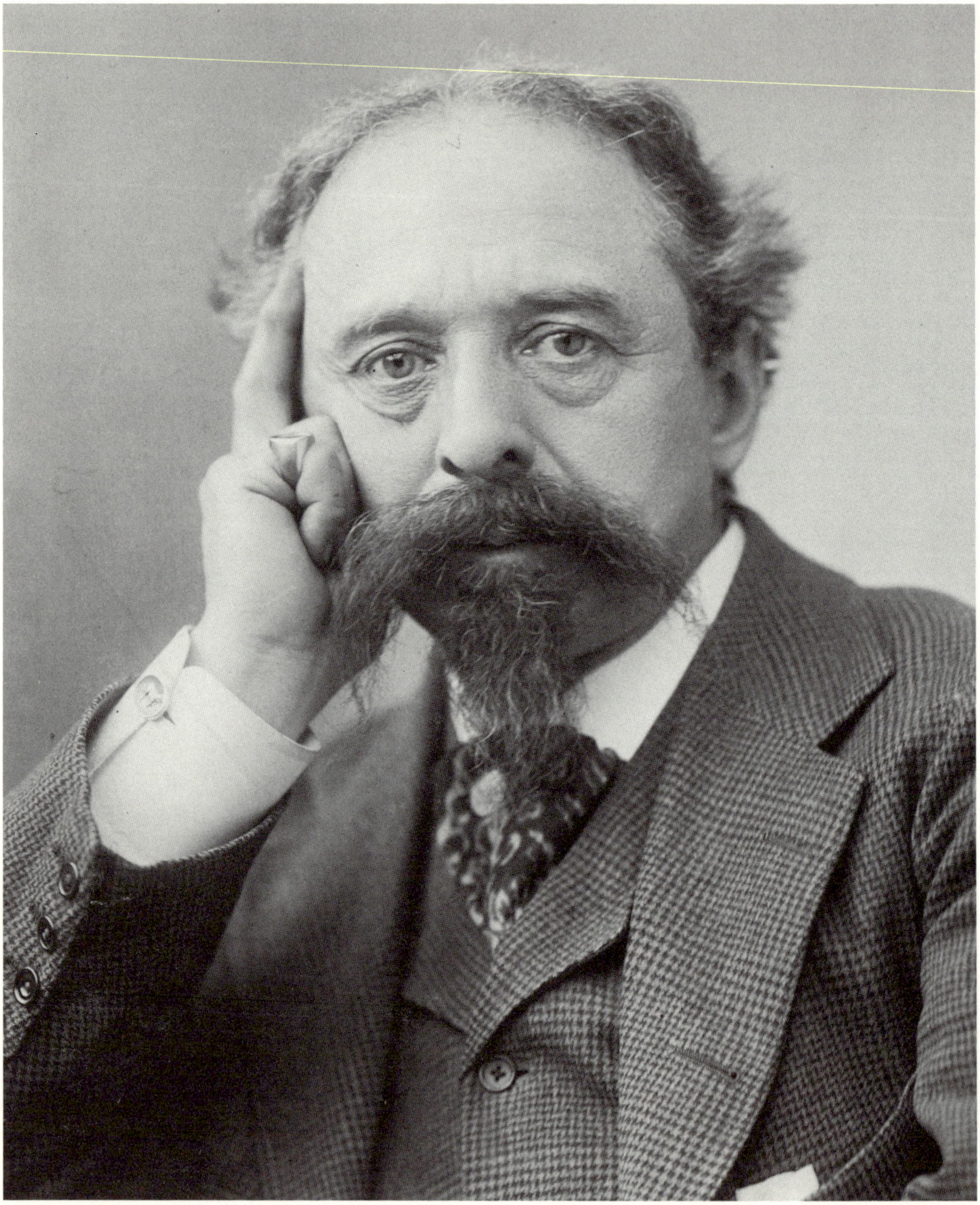

The founding Librarian, James Reed Chadwick, M.D.

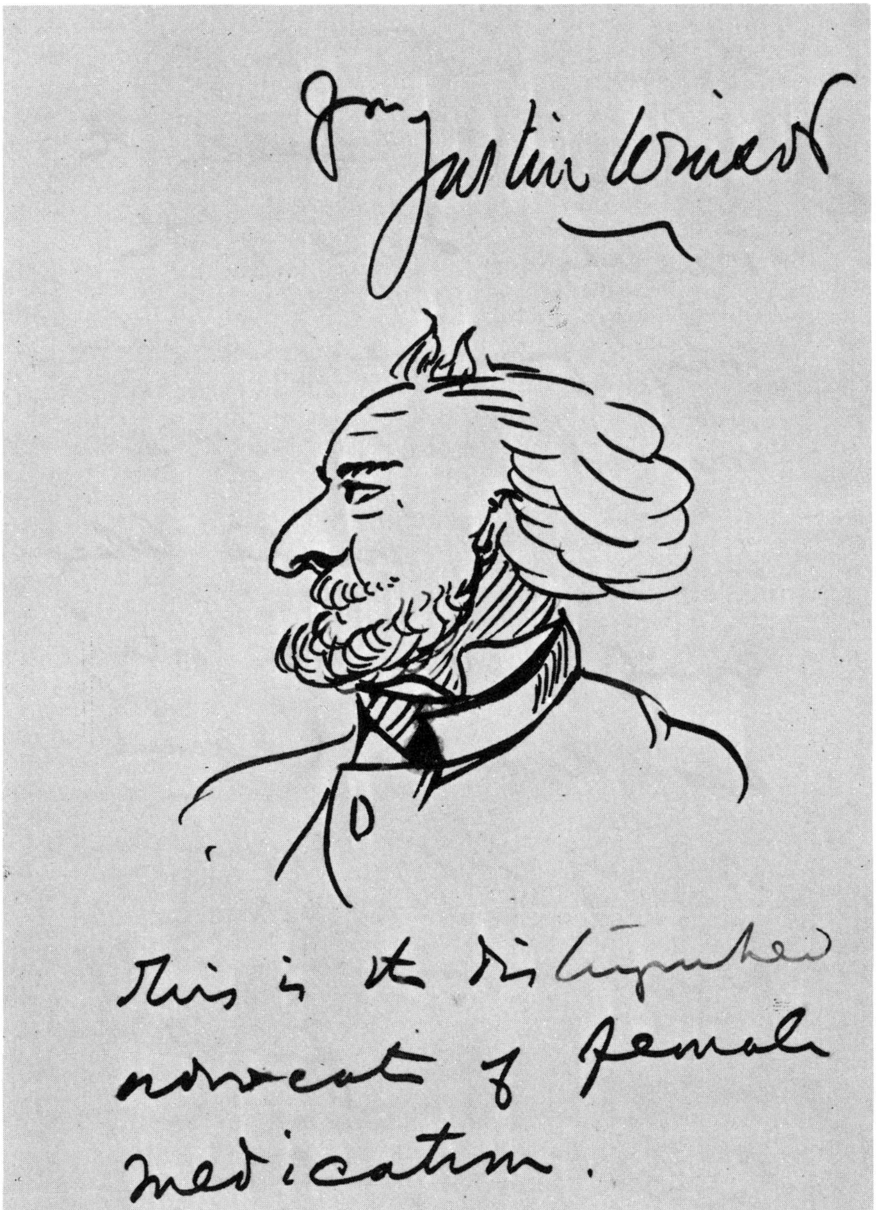

Caricature of his friend Chadwick by Justin Winsor postscripts letter from Cambridge, April 28, 1882, with the caption: "This is the distinguished advocate of female medication."

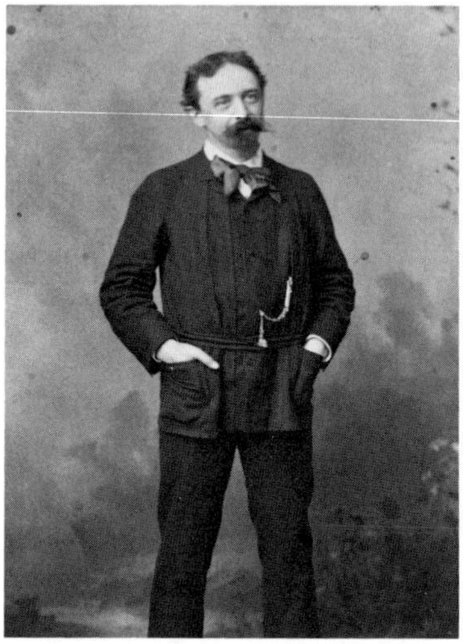

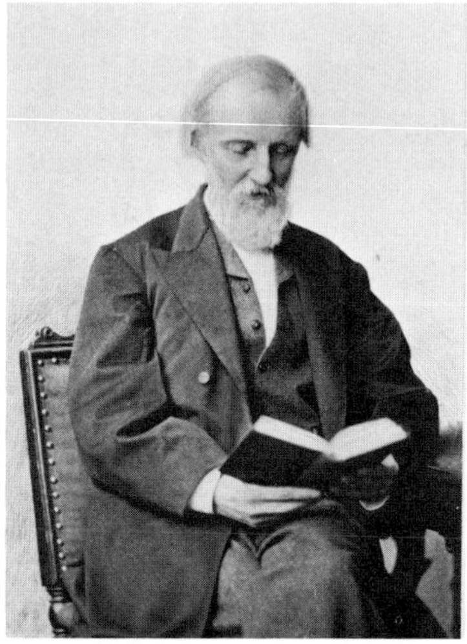

James Reed Chadwick, M.D.

Henry Ingersoll Bowditch, M.D., 1864

Edwin Howard Brigham, M.D.

John Shaw Billings, M.D., about 1890

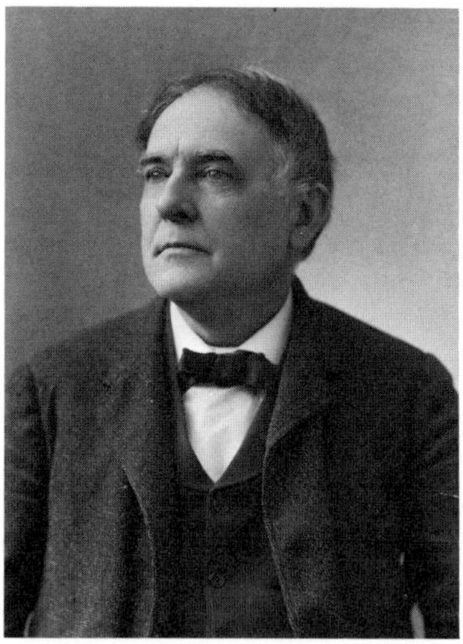

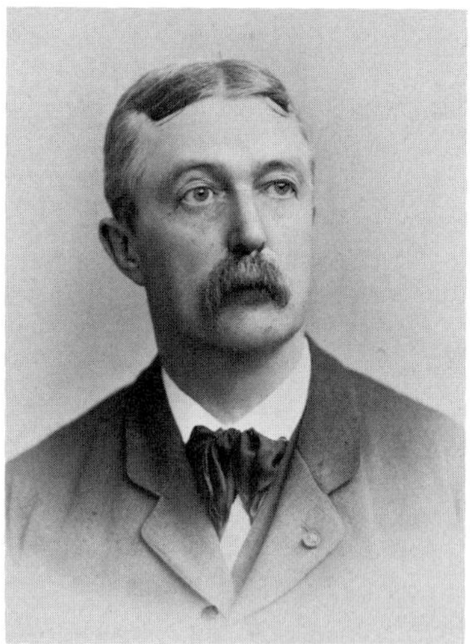

John Shaw Billings was qualmlessly acquisitive in the feeding of his pet project, and it was this October visit to Boston, or perhaps an earlier one (judging from his host's ingenuousness), to which the Army doctor referred later as his *raid* on Chadwick's premises:

I found myself in the library of a physician who had recently returned from Europe, where he had made a collection of books and pamphlets relating to the specialty which he proposed to practice. Among these I observed some old and rare books which I ventured to hint "were peculiarly desirable for the Washington library, where they would be acceptable and be of use to all physicians of the country," etc., etc. The works were promptly placed in my hands, and the doctor proceeded to ransack his shelves, handing down book after book, and asking "if the library had that," or "if it ought not to have that," until a pile had accumulated which actually made me hesitate and feel some embarrassment in accepting,—although by dint of practice I had even at that time acquired a very respectable amount of assurance in such matters. I am glad to say, however, that I allowed no signs of my embarrassment to appear, but succeeded in looking as if matters were merely taking their usual and expected course, and that I carried off everything I could lay my hands on. . . I feel sure that the example which I then set has been faithfully followed, and that your librarian has never forgotten the lesson which must have been strongly impressed upon him as he saw his treasures disappearing.[11]

Chadwick was not the only victim of the audacious visitor from Washington. Billings did not hesitate to invade the *sanctum sanctorum*, the lair of Boston's literary lion, on this or another of his forays, as related by his protegé and biographer, Dr. Fielding H. Garrison:

By means of gifts and exchanges and by ransacking such private collections as were thrown open to him he laboured indefatigably toward completing his collection, obtaining in this way many rare desiderata and filling up many lacunae. Dr. Holmes has humorously described a visit of Billings to his private library in Boston [*sic* Cambridge], how, directly upon entering the room, he swept the shelves with a keen glance, selected the most valuable book in the collection with unerring precision, looked at it a moment, put it back on the shelves, took another look around, and easily found the second book in the scale of values. "Why sir," said Dr. Holmes, "Dr. Billings is a bibliophile of such eminence that I regard him as a positive danger to the owner of a library, if he is ever let loose in it alone."[12]

It was a game two could play, and as must be the case if there is such a thing as progress, the master taught almost better than he knew. It was not long before the temerity of the pupil exceeded even his own, and Billings was writing his Boston friend (the year is unknown) in some slight irritation:

War Department
Surgeon General's Office
Washington. Dec 9th

My dear Chadwick,

The things which you picked out for yourself personally I will send you.

The mass which you picked out for the Library I will not send until you can give a quid pro quo. You might as well have selected our entire stock of duplicates while you were about it, and you must have taken a number of things which you already have.

On the *Exchange* account I think this Library has already a balance to its credit with your Library. A few numbers or volumes to complete particular sets I would let you have, but not the mass you have laid out.

Very sincerely yours
J S Billings[13]

The bound journal collection of the Boston Society for Medical Observation, 911 volumes in all, was Chadwick's working stake in this game of swaps. The Society was to retain ownership of the books and their cases, to insure them, to continue to bind accessions and to retain the right of borrowing for its members. Doctors Buckingham, Wigglesworth and Francis H. Brown, chiefly, toiled with the Librarian to compile a catalogue, and with these cards in hand, Chadwick was, as he put it, "authorized to make a series of raids upon all the private medical libraries of Boston. . . I personally visited every physician in town who was known to have a considerable library, and from these I solicited, and usually obtained, such as I wanted."[14]

The first such library solicited and obtained was the obstetrical collection of upwards of two hundred volumes, amassed by Dr. William Read (HMS 1842), the City Physician and Observation Society member, while engaged in the research for his classic work, *Placenta Praevia: Its History and Treatment*, published in 1861. In the course of exhausting everything on the subject in the Athenaeum's inheritance from the first Boston Medical Library, Read sent abroad for what he could not find in Boston and wound up with most of the standard works on midwifery in existence.[15]

Chadwick next, in January 1876, inveigled from the trustees of the Boston Dispensary, in clouds of dust, the library of the late Dr. John B. Alley (HMS 1844), who had died in 1862; its chief value was in its collection of Sydenham Society publications. Then, for thirty cents each, he purchased 271 bound volumes of the exchanges received for the *Boston Medical and Surgical Journal* from its publisher, David Clapp & Sons. And in April the Medical Improvement Society followed the lead of the Observationists, and the precedent of its predecessor which had created the first medical library seventy years before, and deposited its 474 volumes on the same terms.

The ravages inflicted upon their cherished journals by the brash young raider provoked a deal of muttering among the elders of the twin societies, who feared that Chadwick "was going to turn everything upside down. He seemed, in their eyes, an irrepressible youngster with more zeal than discretion. . . It seems almost incredible that these old societies should have been willing to turn over their books to the charge of an enthusiastic young man and his friends, none of whom had had any library experience."[16] So thought Farlow.

But Chadwick carried all before him, and at the first annual meeting of the Boston Medical Library Association on October 3, 1876, he toted up the booty: 2639 volumes of American and foreign journals, 1445 books in the general library, 404 in the obstetrical section, 3000 pamphlets, 120 journals received regularly by gift, exchange with the *Boston Medical and Surgical Journal* and subscription. . . 133 members. . . solvency, and the recommendation of the executive committee that the dues be dropped from ten to six dollars, an amendment to the by-laws duly adopted. The twenty-six members present re-elected Dr. Holmes and the rest of the slate in disregard of the diffidence he had expressed to Chadwick earlier in the year:

296 Beacon St. Feb 16th, 1876.

Dear Dr Chadwick

I am very happy to subscribe to the Medical Library and may take an interest in it by and by, if it succeeds, as I think it will if your own and others' young blood goes into its veins.

But I cannot consent to be its figure-head, as I was once threatened with being made.

You must get a leader who will keep his traces taut and not have the wheel-horses treading on his heels.

Very truly yours
O W Holmes[17]

Almost everything about this note but the date, which is unmistakable,would lead one to suppose that Holmes had written it before consenting to be the first president in August 1874. Clearly, he had very little to do with the founding of the Library beyond encouraging the younger man and lending his name, rather reluctantly.

Some time during 1876 Dr. William Osler, whose students at McGill University (some of them older than he) affectionately called him "The Baby Professor," paid his first professional visit to the baby library in Boston. He was twenty-seven. Several years later, when Professor of Medicine at Johns Hopkins, he recalled the "kindly interest" of Dr. Brigham on this occasion when, "as a youngster interested in certain clinical subjects to which I could find no reference in our library at McGill, I came to Boston, and I here found what I wanted, and I found moreover a cordial welcome and many friends. It was a small matter I was seeking, but I wished to make it as complete as possible, and I have always felt that this library helped me to a good start."[18]

It was the inception of Osler's lifelong interest in the Library, inspired conceivably by the encouraging puff given the contents of the two rooms in Hamilton Place by Dr. Billings in October : "The medical library of most promise in Boston is that of the Medical Library Association, which, though only one year old, has about three thousand volumes, and will probably rapidly increase."[19]

The legislation incorporating the Boston Medical Library Association on May 7, 1877[20] under the laws of the Commonwealth of Massachusetts was accepted by the members at the annual meeting on October 2, and the by-laws were amended to remove the Librarian from the executive committee and its ex officio chairmanship and empower it to elect one of its own the president of the Library; the committee was henceforth to serve two years, but under no injunction against re-election, meaning self-perpetuation.

Between raiding and cajoling, Dr. Billings had expanded the catalogue entries in the Surgeon General's Library from six hundred in 1865 to over fifty thousand in ten years. Yet the mass of the literature remained an unmapped bibliographic jungle; such paths as had once existed were the more overgrown each passing day with the proliferation of the vines of specialty in this rainy season of the new science. But Billings was an explorer born, and a soldier trained, and in 1876 he plunged into the bush with the publication of his preview to his great work, the *Specimen Fasciculus*; it was a sample of the *Index Medicus* which he had in mind, the monthly guide to current literature which would appear full-blown in 1879, and the *Index Catalogue*, in 1880.

The Washington and Boston medical librarians kept in quite close touch. Each had a stake in the other's progress. . . and duplicates. At the rate the literature was growing, collection without classification meant chaos. Both knew that Billings's struggles to shake down his sytems of indexing and cataloguing contained the key to the future of medical bibliography. The day after the Boston library's incorporation he wrote Chadwick:

Washington D.C.
May 8th 1877.

Dear Doctor

Yours of the 6th rec'd. I have not yet got the classification arranged for the Index, in fact am just beginning to work on it. Each card as it came along was put under the head which seemed most natural, and now I am going over the cards to find out what these heads are, and to condense them if I can. In other words my classification will not be *a priori* but *a posteriori.*

You have my rough classification in pencil on your cards. If you will arrange these alphabetically you will have all that the clerk could give, in fact more, for you must remember that my clerk is not a medical man, and he has no idea as to what would come under gynaecology and what not.

I am afraid my Boston trip must be deferred. I find that I shall probably have to attend the Am Med Ass'n in Chicago in June—and I cannot be absent much—as both my official and Baltimore work are pressing, and cannot be done by deputy.

Yours as always,
J S Billings

P.S. Since writing the above I have discovered a rough draught of what you want—prepared some time ago for a special purpose. It is not at all a complete classification—but a hasty memorandum of card headings—for correction and filling up. Please return it—and pencil on it corrections and additions.

JSB[21]

While plundering the bookeries of his confreres, applying the techniques of Billings to the spoils, practising gynecology, taking a lead in organizing the department at City Hospital, teaching at the Medical School and joining with his father-in-law in founding the American Gynecological Society, Jim Chadwick found time in 1877 to accept appointment to the Boston Public Library's examining committee of five citizens-at-large designated each year by the trustees to inspect the premises and report back on their condition and welfare. The Boston City Council had chosen this particular year to meddle in the affairs of the library by adopting an order which reduced several salaries, not the least of which was that of the excellent Librarian, Justin Winsor. The examining committee examined this political interference in a supposedly sacrosanct department of the city, and Chadwick composed its report castigating the politicians and urging in the strongest terms that the library be placed on an independent status. This step was taken the next year in the Act of Incorporation of 1878, but not before Winsor had resigned to accept President Eliot's canny invitation to be the Librarian of Harvard College.

Before 1877 was out, two years of this kind of explosive energy from Chadwick had overwhelmed the two small rooms at 5 Hamilton Place. The rejects from the shelves lay in heaps by the hundreds on the floor, while three promised collections were of necessity held back. There were the eight hundred volumes recently willed by Dr. Edward H. Clarke, Professor of Materia Medica Emeritus at Harvard and a co-founder with Bowditch of the revived Observation Society; next in the waiting line were the many rare books which Doctors George Brune Shattuck and Frederick Cheever Shattuck had persuaded their father, Dr. George Cheyne Shattuck, Jr., the recently retired Professor of the Theory and Practice of Medicine, to donate to the new library; finally was the extensive collection (ever the hand of Chadwick) which the Gynecological Society of Boston had voted to deposit. Duplicates by the thousands, numbering complete files of the leading Anglo-American journals, awaited space and the marshalling energy of the Librarian, who dreamed of sending them forth to circulate into every corner of the Commonwealth for the good uses of the profession. It was a wish long in the fulfillment. Too often readers could scarely find chair room, while medical students were flat out of luck, barred from the premises for lack of space.

Starting from scratch, and with the most anemic of resources, Chadwick and his raids and seductions in two years made Boston's new medical library with its eight thousand volumes the sixth largest in the United States behind Billings's Surgeon General's (40,000), the College of Physicians (19,000) and Pennsylvania Hospital (12,500) in Philadelphia, the New York Hospital (10,000) and the Boston Public Library (10,000).

Dr. Holmes must have been relieved that the dashing fellow was on *his* side. If Billings was a positive danger to the owner of a private library, Jim was a pied piper let loose. Trouble was, where to put all those books he tootled off their keepers' shelves and out the door, to march mesmerized in his train?

4

Mrs. Howe's Kitchen

1878 · 1889

After two years of tumescence the Boston Medical Library was ripe to burst from its secluded cocoon in the shadow of the Park Street Church. By late in 1877 Dr. Chadwick was casting about for larger quarters. Meandering across the Common and browsing Boylston Street where many of the doctors had their offices, his Bohemian spirit paused happily beneath a row of baleful bay windows in another blind alley, Boylston Place, remembered by Dr. Farlow as a damp and cheerless cul-de-sac "of rather unsavory reputation later on." One of these bays overhung the recessed stoop of number 19, a three-story brick front home from which the recently deceased humanitarian, Dr. Samuel Gridley Howe, and his literary wife, Julia Ward Howe of *Battle Hymn of the Republic* fame, had some years since escaped. It was now a boarding house and just right for a medical library—dignified and somewhat doleful.

Dr. Holmes, who must have held forth in Mrs. Howe's parlor more than once, and the executive committee were agreeably impressed. On February 25, 1878 they mounted an appeal to the profession, framed by the Librarian, for $5000 to secure a mortgage. Most recently a boarding house, the Howe residence needed hardly an alteration to be turned into a library, they declared. Moreover, "in seeking to acquire possession of this house, the Association has a still greater object in view; that of ultimately establishing a permanent home for all the societies devoted to the study of medicine and the kindred sciences in this city." To this end it was proposed to build a meeting hall on the street level. Here is the first suggestion that the Boston Medical Library should expand into an academy of medicine.[1]

The response emboldened the officers on March 9 to go after $15,000. By the end of the month a purchase price of $13,000 had been agreed upon; C. P. Putnam and F. I. Knight were appointed the building committee and the well-known Boston architect Henry Van Brunt was engaged. Simultaneously, the treasurer was warning that because the dues of more than fifty members remained unpaid, he hadn't the funds to meet his bills; he was told to hire a bill collector if he had to.

Nineteen Boylston Place was shouldered, out of the usual numerical sequence, between number 20, which was Hopkinson's Private School for Boys, and number 18, the dwelling of the late historian John Lothrop Motley, as staid as the other was boisterous, occupied since 1870 by the Boston Library Society.[2]

Two doors away, Mrs. George Sturgis had bought number 17 and moved in with her two daughters in 1858 after the death of her husband. Subsequently she married Agustin Ruiz de Santayana in Spain and returned to Boston in 1872 with him, her girls and a son of six, George Santayana. On what the philosopher in the hindsight of his memoirs viewed as the ill advice of her brother-in-law, James Sturgis, his mother purchased a new house on the water side of Beacon Street, but instead of selling number 17, put it out to rent. His Uncle James had argued that Boylston Place, "genteelly retired in the '50's, had become unsuitable for two young girls about to enter society; several of the houses had become boarding houses, or something even worse. On the other hand business was flooding Boylston Street, just at the head of Boylston Place, and could not fail to run down that little slope and flood Boylston Place also. Let my mother move from Boylston Place but not sell her house, No. 17, because what with the business flowing down (in his imagination) from the busy street above, and the boarding houses requiring just such central but retired spots to flourish in, that property would prove a bonanza: the rent could be increased with every new lease." Number 17 was still in the family's hands (where it would remain for some years) when Dr. Chadwick took his fancy to what Santayana remembered disagreeably as "a disreputable back alley. . . I call it disreputable dramatically, as my mother would have called it if she had understood: but it was simply Bohemian. Vercelli's Italian restaurant was there in my time, and the Tavern Club, the only club I ever belonged to in Boston; and I frequented both, until they became stuffy and tiresome. . ."[3]

In the Medical Library's conversion of number 19 which soon got under way, the old Howe parlor with the bay on the second floor became the main reading room. Dr. Brigham and periodicals occupied a smaller room to the rear. The largest on the third floor was rented to the American Statistical Association for its library on vital statistics and insanity; the remainder was used for cataloguing. The Brighams lived in the closer confines of the fourth floor, really more of an attic, rent-free;

the assistant librarian's salary of eight hundred dollars a year was considered emolument enough.

The meeting hall was something else. With a seating capacity of a hundred and twenty, it was *nonpareil* the wonder of Boylston Place, and the herniation of it from a town house twenty-seven feet wide into the back of a lot sixty feet deep was viewed by the responsible parties as a brilliant technological breakthrough. To manage it, Henry Van Brunt miniaturized, after a fashion, another of his *chef d'oeuvres*, Harvard's Memorial Hall, by ripping out most of the first floor, breaking through the rear wall and inserting an iron beam at the second floor level, then tearing down Mrs. Howe's kitchen ell in the back yard and erecting a two-story windowless structure over the basement and out into the yard. The flat roof of the hall beyond the house was fitted with a sizeable skylight for illumination.

Access to this truncated temple of Aesculapius was by a broad flight of steps, each deep enough to set chairs on, which descended from what remained of the Howe's front hall. Sheer cliffs of bookcases rose eighteen and a half feet from floor to ceiling, divided by a catwalk reached up a spiral stair. Thus was barred the portly browser from the heights. Not so, however, below, where early meeting attendants misplaced books or left them lying about while awaiting the call of the chair; to confound such absentmindedness, a net curtain was hung in front of the shelves which were within reach of the floor, weighted at the bottom by iron rods, but it frustrated Dr. Brigham more than anyone and was discarded after a few months. The rails of the galleries groaned with Chadwick's collected portraits of medical dignitaries, the important and the less so. Benjamin Waterhouse and his rival, John Collins Warren, in grimy plaster from the shoulders up, stared down unblinkingly from their perches at the gallery corners above the chairman's desk, beneath a brace of Van Brunt's reassuring trusses. Other reminders that all is temporal were stationed about the hall. The general atmosphere of the place was moderated from a tall, dark cabinet which stood, a deathly sentinel's box, below Dr. Warren; it was occupied by the Library's taciturn reference skeleton, Jake.

The twenty-eight gas jets which shed their blaze upon the nighttime deliberations of the profession were concealed within the double skylight (for that is what it was), where the warmth they generated was supposed to provide the final pull for a ventilating and heating arrangement that was in no way out of character with the edifice. As there was nowhere else for it, the boiler room was put behind the stairs descending broadly to the hall. Steam pipes were run under the steps inside long iron boxes. Adjustable vents through the risers of the stairs were controlled by a system of levers. At the opposite end of the hall, behind the rostrum, rose a bank of panelled flue boxes against the wall (as if concealing organ pipes) which vented into the overhead space within the double skylight.

Outside air drawn in through the boiler room by the escaping heat of the gas jets aloft was commanded to pass obediently at a designed velocity of two feet a second across the steam pipes under the stairs and into the meeting place, in quantities measured by the vent levers. It was then expected to move draughtlessly among the audience, in defiance of every high school physics text, before entering the intakes at the floor level of the flue boxes on the opposite wall. Thence it was to take its leave by way of the escape hatches above the skylight and into the Boston night, carrying with it the undesirable byproducts of human metabolism at a velocity of no less than three feet per second.

Much attention had been given to this ingenious contrivance, with all its subtleties and refinements, by architect Van Brunt and Doctors Putnam, Knight and Chadwick. To get the benefit of expert consultation, they submitted the thermodynamics to Dr. Edward Cowles, a psychiatrist at City Hospital who was said to be an expert on this sort of problem. Probably because Dr. John Shaw Billings was at the time involved in the design of Johns Hopkins Hospital, Chadwick asked his advice too. Writing from Washington on June 24, 1878, Billings suggested a few minor modifications in the heating and ventilating setup and counseled:

> If you use steam I would advise a warm plate somewhere in the Hall where wet feet can be dried. This had best be a box containing a steam coil— and filled with sand covered with a movable plate. . . You should distinctly understand that while .10 percent of CO^2 may be called a permissible amount of impurity in the sense that in two hours or so it will produce no marked bad effects except headache in the more sensitive, yet it should not be considered a permissible impurity in a hall arranged for *Medical Men* in the *City of Boston*. . .[4]

Admirable, proudly pronounced Dr. Putnam in his report for the building committee. However, performance fell short of a conception whose naiveté, not to mention its presumption, both astounds and amuses. "Dr. Brigham always had great difficulty in regulating the covers of the steam-pipe boxes under the steps," smiled Farlow, "and the general effect was, hot air around the head and arctic breezes about the legs of the audience. The system seemed to try to make hot air from the steam-pipes go down to the floor where it was needed and stay there."[5]

The new home of the Boston Medical Library Association, assuredly ample for generations to come, was dedicated on December 3, 1878.[6] The galleries were hung with a loan collection of seventy-two portraits of late medical men of Massachusetts, many of which were later donated, all gathered by Chadwick. The fascinating hall was packed. At one end the steam-pipe boxes held forth, at the other, the speakers, led off by President Holmes, who, after a charming explication on the delights and uses of books, singular and in the aggregate, and of libraries, personal (his own) and institutional, complimented whimsically (as related in the previous chapter) the young men led by Chadwick who had finally brought to pass in Boston what the old men had longed for. Then he brought his most serious concern to bear on what he recognized as the Library's pressing contemporary goal: to make readily available to the profession the expanding array of the world's periodical literature. But how, without an index?

> Who wants a lock without a key, a ship without a rudder, a binnacle without a compass, a check without a signature, a greenback without a goldback behind it?. . . [Journals] heap themselves into chaotic piles and bundles which are worse than useless, taking up a great deal of room, and frightening everything away but mice and mousing antiquarians, or possibly at long intervals some terebrating specialist. Arranged, bound, indexed, all these at once become accessible and valuable.

Indexing, in the long view of Dr. Holmes, "is the special need of our time in medical literature." He looked to Washington and the Surgeon General's Library to show the way.

> That great and growing collection of fifty thousand volumes is under the eye and hand of a librarian who knows books and how to manage them. For libraries are the standing armies of civilization, and an army is but a mob without a general who can organize and marshal it so as to make it effective. The "Specimen Fasciculus of a Catalogue of the National Medical Library," prepared under the direction of Dr. Billings, the librarian, would have excited the admiration of Haller, the master scholar in medical science of the last century, or rather of the profession in all centuries, and if carried out as it is begun will be to the nineteenth all and more than all that the three Bibliothecae—Anatomica, Chirurgica, and Medicinae-Practicae—were to the eighteenth century.

Dr. Billings was on hand and remarked that the Boston library had outgrown his advice—"You have already reached that stage of development when you are having practical experience of the truth of that maxim which should always be in the mind of the librarian, namely, 'Unto him that hath shall be given.' "

President Eliot of Harvard and his librarian, Justin Winsor, brought greetings, and so did Dr. Chadwick's father-in-law, Dr. George H. Lyman, now president of the Massachusetts Medical Society. The program concluded with the blessing of the Library's patriarchal vice president who had succeeded upon Dr. Buckingham's death in 1876, Dr. Henry I. Bowditch, just into his threescore and ten, evoking his almost lifelong dream of the reality then under dedication. Characteristically, he threw the credit to the younger men. "I have admired the tact and ability with which they have overcome opposition, and I now feel disposed to thank them most heartily, not merely for myself, but for the community at large, for the profession of the present day and that of the far future."

Of course no one present could have an inkling of how sensitized would become the synapse inadvertently activated in Boylston Place by the emissaries from Cambridge. President Eliot expressed the amiable hope that the Medical School might arrange with the Library to admit students to privileges, while Justin Winsor suggested building a passageway from the Boston Public Library around the corner on Boylston Street and ventured "I think that the time will come when the two libraries and that of the Medical School will be brought into intimate relations."

Nonetheless, a week later the executive committee voted to bar dogs from the new building and in four more, on January 18, 1879, reaffirmed the ban on medical students. . . "it is inexpedient at the present time to take any steps looking to the admission of the students of the Harvard Medical School as a body."

Creature of Harvard faculty and alumni as the Library was, the closed-door policy against the students en masse probably reflects less of hauteur than of uneasiness lest the pleasant and relaxed new quarters be overrun by the unquellable and unquenchable.

The fund campaign had brought in something over $10,000, which, with a mortgage of $8000, secured the Howe house and built the hall with its gadgetry, leaving, nevertheless, a floating debt of $4000. Van Brunt's trusses still vibrated to the dedicatory plaudits as the officers wrestled with the bill. Meeting in Dr. Wigglesworth's office at 108 Boylston Street on December 14,[7] they decided to go ahead with a scheme "for appointing a physician in each ward to canvass the ward, or, when the above measure is from any cause undesirable, canvassing by missionaries." They also voted that the hall should be "Jackson Hall" and "a first-rate portrait of the late Dr. James Jackson shall be painted and hung there in consideration of the sum of $10,000." A week later Dr. Chadwick reported back that there was little hope of raising that kind of money for a portrait (a wildly unrealistic proposition in the first place for an association already $4000 in the hole), and the idea was dropped. With it faded all enthusiasm for naming the hall after Dr. Jackson.

It was less difficult to keep the hall filled. The Observation, Improvement, Massachusetts and Suffolk District medical societies were invited to make it their meeting place, and all accepted. The Observation and Mass Medical societies agreed to pay $125 and $150 annual rent for the privilege.

Some profit must also have been derived from the decision to permit Dr. Brigham to sell professionally the vaccine points developed and produced by that most remarkable general practitioner of Roxbury, Dr. Henry Austin Martin (HMS 1845). A spontaneous case of cowpox in Beaugency, France, in 1866 had been the means of reintroducing a strong virus by way of a heifer and of obviating continued use of increasingly risky humanized strains. Martin brought Beaugency virus to America in 1870, and in 1877 unveiled the modern method of standardization and vaccination.[8] It was the same year that he came up with the rubber bandage for the treatment of leg ulcers which bears his name.

For his pains Dr. Martin was abused. "I gave them every aid in my power freely, frankly, and fully, and was repaid by ingratitude, slander, and an effort, as futile as it was earnest and persistent, to rob me of the scrap of professional honor and reputation I had worked so hard to win and deserve, in introducing and firmly establishing in America a system which has already conferred infinite though hardly fully appreciated blessings."[9]

The vaccinator was a surgeon veteran of the Civil War, a friend of the Library, a booklover and medical historian, besides which—as the foregoing example of his prose style intimates—he relished the lists. Dr. Brigham remembered his jousts with Dr. B. E. Cotting, who "had a forceful personality and assumed to rule the Norfolk District Medical Society but was antagonized at every turn by Dr. Henry Austin Martin, the introducer of pure animal vaccine. Every meeting of the district society was attended by breezy arguments and drew a large attendance for the fun. Dr. Martin was a fine looking man, a most fluent speaker, eloquent, witty, pathetic. Of Celtic origin, he played on the heart strings and almost made Dr. Cotting appear to be unfair, selfish, dogmatic and a near villain."[10]

The Beaugency vaccine points "were considered to be the best and also absolutely fresh, being delivered by Dr. Martin's agent directly to the library. This business was continued for many years and was a source of satisfaction to the doctors."[11]

Oddly enough, the most useful, remunerative and far-reaching innovation of the early years (and no more germane to its bibliographic purpose than the sale of vaccine points) was set in motion with the designation of Frederick C. Shattuck and Charles P. Putnam as a subcommittee of the executive committee on July 12, 1879 to provide for the registration of nurses at the Library. Shattuck was then thirty-one, a *brillant* if not a dilletante, and rather bored with practice.[12] Putnam, three years older, a founder of the Library, more serious in outlook, was elected the same year the first president of the Associated Charities of Boston and was on his way to renown and indeed reverence as an advancer of good causes in social medicine.

Nurses available for home duty had been listed in the Boston Directory as early as 1830, *sans* addresses. By 1850 this helpful information had been added, but it was no great relief to patients and physicians, whose plight in Boston, as elsewhere, was described by Dr. Shattuck in the first report of the subcommittee:

> . . . Any person to whose lot it fell to try to secure a competent nurse for a case of sudden illness was compelled to get a long list of nurses from a physician or friend, and often to spend hours of precious time in driving about the city before a nurse could be found; and then, too frequently, the employer had to put up with what was to be had rather than what was desired.[13]

The Directory followed naturally on the organization at the Massachusetts General Hospital in 1873 of the Boston Training School for Nurses, the third of its kind in the United States. Dr. Putnam was a founder of that important adjunct, with various American admirers of Florence Nightingale including Miss Mary Anne Wales, its first secretary, who had been largely responsible with Miss Sarah Cabot and Mrs. Samuel Parkman for implementing the idea of formal nursing education which had originated in the Industrial Committee of the Woman's Education Association of Boston, ever on the lookout for new occupations for self-supporting females. Miss Wales, Miss A. P. Dixwell and Mrs. M. R. Towne were identified by Dr. Shattuck in his first report as the "public-spirited and experienced ladies. . . to whose self-sacrificing and unwearied labors a large measure of the success of the Directory is due." Dr. Brigham agreed to serve as Registrar. The remaining essential, one of the earliest telephones in Boston (number 113), was installed in October. In November of 1879 the Directory for Nurses opened for business at the Boston Medical Library with a list of sixty. Shattuck believed it to be "the first of its kind ever established. . . [It] will doubtless lead to the formation of similar ones in other large cities."[14]

Within two years the Directory was listing 412 nurses—366 women earning eight to twenty dollars a week, and forty-six men twenty to thirty-five (!). Seventy-five (whether of both sexes the record does not specify) were graduates of reputable training schools, chiefly those of the MGH, City Hospital and the New England Hospital for Women and Children.

The agency assessed physician and family references provided by nurses seeking work, and if they met the standards of the committee, listed and updated them. Besides training, qualifications, specialty, rates and so on, applicants were required to state "whether he or she is willing to take meals in the kitchen." The registration fee for nurses quickly rose from fifty cents to three dollars. Employers were charged a dollar during the day and two at night, for Dr. Brigham was furnished with a night bell as well as phone and was on call around the clock. For another dollar, families could have the nurse "laid down at their doors." The fee for finding a wet nurse was five dollars.[15]

Miss Sara E. Parsons, former Superintendent of Nurses at the MGH, wrote of the Directory at Boylston Place in her history of the training school published in 1922:

> The first registry for nurses was established at the Boston Medical Library, and managed, to a considerable extent, after the customs of an employment bureau. There are nurses still living who remember their interviews with the Registrar [Dr. Brigham], who asked them to read a little from a book so that he could estimate their educational qualification and their fitness for entertaining the patient by reading aloud. . . For some years it was stated in the circulars that the nurse was to eat in the kitchen with the servants. Eventually this was recognized as an unwise arrangement, as well as objectionable to the nurses, and was so stated in an admirable lecture on private duty given to the students in 1886 by Dr. William Richardson. . .
>
> A superintendent in New York who was interested in starting a registry there in the early eighties, wrote to the Registrar in Boston concerning the details of organizing it. He wrote back not to start one, that she would hate herself and everybody else before she got through. Thus one suspects that the registry had its own troubles.[16]

Troubles and all, within five years the income the Directory for Nurses turned in to the Boston Medical Library so far exceeded any other single source of revenue, including dues, as to stifle the groans of members who complained vainly about the bustle and rustle which unavoidably attended the furnishing of 1315 nurses throughout the Boston area and in fact New England over a twelve-month period.[17]

The overnight success of the Directory, combined with the reduction of the $4000 floating debt by three-quarters and the growth of the Library encouraged the executive committee in October 1881 to tackle its remaining indebtedness of some $9000. Dr. Holmes again headed the appeal for "a new subscription of fifteen thousand dollars for the purpose of cancelling the entire debt, making some pressing and long-neglected alterations and repairs, and having a small fund for binding and for buying new books, as soon as issued." The officers breezily assured the members that "with this sum we feel that the Library Association will be established on so lasting a basis as to preclude the necessity of appeals for pecuniary assistance in the future."[18]

The genius of John Shaw Billings began paying off with the appearance of the *Index Medicus* in 1879, the *Index Catalogue* a year later. The compass recommended for the binnacle by Dr. Holmes was at hand. Now steersmen were needed, and American medicine could fairly begin the voyage on the referential seas of the new science. . . in Boston's case, a steerswoman in the person of Mrs. Elizabeth J. Collins. Dr. Chadwick engaged her as a part-time cataloguer in 1880, and Dean Calvin Ellis of Harvard Medical School at first paid her salary. She would remain on the job for forty-two years.

At fourteen Mrs. Collins had been forced by her father's death to quit school. After a year she landed a job at the Boston Public Library, where she remained for eleven years until her marriage to Thomas Collins in 1876. Her husband died in 1879, and the widow returned to the Public Library, resuming charge of the medical section under the direction of Justin Winsor. It was said that Mrs. Collins knew more than anyone else around about the cataloging of the medical literature because mainly she invented her own system. Such a useful person attracted the interest of Chadwick, and gradually he hired her away until in 1881 she was full time at Boylston Place.

To Mrs. Collins the *Indices* were heaven sent, and Dr. Billings the sender. Soon she made his acquaintance through Chadwick, and for years after received the benefit of his advice and not infrequently advance notice of yet uncatalogued items by way of this inside track. The main line to the Surgeon General's Library was kept well traveled between the terminals of "The Washington Box" in Boston which was reserved for items that might be of interest to the national library (with a similar box, probably, at the other end), and Chadwick's regular pilgrimages to Washington every few months to mend his fences and swap duplicates.

Mrs. Collins was a legendary worker, but she could never pitch the fork as fast as the Librarian sowed and swung the scythe, and by 1884—though she had catalogued nearly all that she had come upon four years earlier—success had bred so much success that the harvest lay in windrows all about. There were the Clarke and Shattuck libraries already mentioned, released now to the supposedly safer quarters as promised. Then there were seven hundred volumes collected by the late Dean Ellis, the medical books of the Roxbury Athenaeum, the library of more than four hundred bequeathed by Dr. Thomas Buckminster Curtis (whom Dr. Coll Warren regarded as a walking catalogue of the surgical literature),[19] and most unexpectedly in 1880 the large library and portrait of Dr. Samuel Wheeler Wyman of Newburyport, who had died in 1867, given by his maiden daughters.

Dr. Wyman opened practice in Ipswich after his graduation from Harvard Medical School in 1818, and when he shifted down to Newburyport after three years of it he quite literally took his office with him, to the corner of State and Temple streets, to be exact. This qualified him as the butt for one of a collection of contemporary "epitaphs" contrived by a gossipsome lady of that genteel old seaport:

Here lies Dr. Wyman,
That snug little shyman,
Whose house always traveled when he did;
But he might have been kept
In the room where he slept,
For a closer grave never was needed.[20]

(The investment of shelf and wall in Dr. Wyman was harvested when the will of Miss Ellen Brewer Wyman was read in 1913. She left the residue of her estate to the Library in his memory—some $92,000 in cash and several commercial properties on State Street in Newburyport, the old doctor having got shut out of his traveling house before his last move, after all. The Library managed the real estate and finally sold it in 1922 and 1923 to its considerable profit and the immense relief of the officers.)

The quite staggering autograph holdings of the Boston Medical Library were built on Robert C. Winthrop's gift in 1879 of letters relating to medical problems received between 1643 and 1663 by his forebears, John Winthrop, father and son, governors of Massachusetts and Connecticut. The earliest of these was "Receipts to cure various Disorders For my worthy friend Mr. Wintrop," dated May 6, 1643 from Edward Stafford at London. Robert Winthrop was president of the Massachusetts Historical Society when he turned this correspondence over to Dr. Holmes, who considered the most outlandish of Stafford's compounds to be his *black powder against ye plague, small-pox, purples, all sorts of feavers, pyson, either by way of prevention or after infections.* "Formidable to the imagination," grunted the emeritus. "This is made by burning toads to charcoal, and reducing this to powder. It belongs to that list of abominations which disgraced the old pharmacopias. . ."[21] Not long after the Winthrop gift, the statistician Dr. Edward Jarvis of Boston presented the Library with his collection of almost two thousand letters received during sixty years of correspondence. To its tenant, the American Statistical Association, he gave his own statistical library, which probably helped to push it from the premises in 1886 for lack of space.

As autographs accumulated, Dr. Chadwick (who added several hundred letters himself) embarked bravely but perfectly hopelessly on the project of having them properly mounted. To this gratuitous labor he enlisted Dr. and Mrs. J. H. S. Fogg of South Boston as well as several of his female patients, "an occupation which has proved of great therapeutic value to the persons thus engaged."[22]

Harvard Medical School by autumn of 1883 was about to abandon the old on North Grove Street for the new on lower Boylston Street which President Eliot's dynamism had funded and built. It proved to be the occasion again to ask whether the time had arrived to admit students to the privilege of the Medical Library Association. Conferences were held from which emerged the suggestion that as far as Harvard was concerned the problem could be solved quite nicely by the *Library* moving to the *School*. . . a proposition which the executive committee declined as "disadvantageous to the best interests of the Association." In December the Medical School moved proudly into its Gothic monstrosity in the Back Bay at the corner of Boylston and Exeter streets and the issue of student privileges remained unresolved.

But early in 1884 the rejected suitor was back on the doorstep at 19 Boylston Place, now trying to woo away one of the tenants, the Massachusetts Medical Society, whose officers decided it should stay where it was but pointedly reminded their landlord that "the present condition of the hall is uncomfortable and has been objected to by a large number of the councilors." Their siren hopes dashed, the medical faculty opened a library for the students in the new building and arranged an exchange between the School's older periodicals and books and the Library's duplicates.

The uncomfortable condition of the hall had already come under the scrutiny of the officers, who had to admit that there was something *defective* about the thermodynamics and called in Professor S. H. Wooldridge of the Massachusetts Institute of Technology to see what, if anything, could be done during the summer of 1884.

Fortunately, a delightful reminiscence of the Medical Library in its earlier Boylston Place days has been preserved by the pen of Mrs. Ethel Leatherbee, who was the daughter of Dr. and Mrs. Brigham, adopted by the members as "the library baby," and very nearly the same age as her subject:[23]

Boylston Place was at the time a most desirable residential district. No. 18, the former home of the historian, J. L. Motley, was occupied by the Boston Library Society, No. 17 by the Misses Dabney, No. 21 by the Misses Dexter, No. 1 by Eliot Clark, son of the Unitarian divine, James Freeman Clark, and to No. 4 across the street, soon came the Tavern Club. . . Dr. Howe's dwelling was made over for the library, the first floor and basement being thrown together to form the first subterranean hall in Boston; the second floor and part of the third were set apart for library purposes, and the remainder made into an apartment for the resident librarian and his family, the kitchen and dining room being most curiously located on the top floor in order that the odor of plebeian victuals might not invade the fastidious nostrils of Boston's medicos. . .

I remember well Dr. Oliver Wendell Holmes and Henry Ingersoll Bowditch, who encouraged me shamelessly to steal from our apartments above, to wander in the sacred realms below. They had always some charming story to tell to the little girl, or something toothsome to produce from their capacious pockets. I remember the Autocrat of the Breakfast Table as a slight, short little gentleman, generally dressed in black, who had great bushy eyebrows that he "wiggled" for my delectation.

The great surgeon, Dr. Henry J. Bigelow, with his beautiful, long Dundreary whiskers, was at that time considered the handsomest man in Boston; but more striking, to my childish fancy, was the elegant Dr. James R. Chadwick, first librarian of the society, who wore Norfolk jackets, Windsor ties and a mustache and imperial à la Napoleon III, and who used to dazzle Boylston Place by arriving in his dogcart, the only one in town, with a gold-mounted harness and a pair of dock-tailed cobbs. [Mrs. Leatherbee subsequently corrected herself and thought the driver of the dogcart was probably Dr. George Haven.][24]

Other celebrities were Dr. Reginald Heber Fitz, first to proclaim the lurking dangers in the vermiform appendix; Dr. Robert Hooper, discoverer of the baleful adenoids which have made the fortune of many a specialist since his day,[25] and the great Henry Martin, who established the first cow-pox barns in the country, as a source of animal virus, and distributed the virus on ivory points wrapped in oiled silk. It was Dr. Henry Martin himself who decorated my baby arm with a vaccination scar as large as a silver cartwheel.

I heard of all the new wrinkles in medical progress within those walls, and distinctly remember a long argument between several distinguished doctors on the truth or falsity of the new "germ theory," in which Dr. Philip Knapp was the chief advocate of the new notion.

But, naturally, with the morbidity of childhood, it was the pathological exhibits which made the deepest impression upon me. I remember vividly going into the great hall and coming upon a large platterful of human eyes, which stared at me uncannily. Dr. Ernest Cushing often proudly displayed to his confreres enormous tumors he had removed, while amputated limbs or disembodied organs were always lying about.

Dr. Brigham, Mrs. Leatherbee's father, recalled that as part of his duties as assistant librarian "I was in attendance at every meeting, sitting in the rear of the hall so that I might call out any physician present, if he were wanted by his patients, and to look out for things generally. In a short time I had learned to know every man by the back of his head as well as by his face. The meetings of a clinical character often had piles of tumors and pathological material heaped on the table near the presiding officer's desk for demonstration. Subsequently it was a part of my duty to see that cremation under the boiler took place."[26] His daughter continues:

> Then, too, I always enjoyed unofficially the suppers of the Medical Society. In those happy days catering was an art in which Caterer Tufts was not excelled. There were enormous piles of every sort of salad, large dishes of scalloped oysters, mountains of hearty sandwiches, ice cream in gallon moulds, cases of beer piled high in the corners, and long churchwarden pipes.
>
> Lurking on the stairway in not too discreet secrecy, I was generally taken in tow by dear old Dr. Warner or some other kindly gentleman and stuffed to the limit. Or, if parental watch was too vigilant for such escapades, I took my station below the niche of the plaster cast of the Venus de Medici, where black-dress-suited henchmen of Caterer Tufts smuggled tidbits to me.
>
> One of my most constant friends of those happy days was "Jake" the skeleton, who resided in a green-baize lined box in the hall, next to the rostrum. It was a great social asset to be able to introduce Jake to my schoolmates, who shivered deliciously in approaching his retreat, and must screw up their courage to the very limit to timidly shake his rattling hand.

Perhaps, too, the perquisites of Ethel Brigham's paramedical status among her schoolmates in what to her was *a most desirable residential district* and to George Santayana *a disreputable back alley* included the mantle shed by his older half sister, Susana Sturgis, when their mother moved away in 1861. Susana evidently had informed her brother that "she was the Captain of all the children that played in the street; and if this practice seems not very genteel, we must remember that in Boston, local society was both select and democratic, given an acceptable quarter of the town; and that, as Boylston Place ran downhill, it afforded in winter an irresistible chance for 'coasting,' that is, for tobogganing with single or even with double or longer sleds."[27]

At the center of it all was Jim Chadwick, elegant to childish eyes, but something less and something more in those of his friend Billings, who wrote him from Washington: "Take my advice and put aside that blouse of yours. It's comfortable and artistic but it's not professional—and I heard the other day in the course of a brief discussion on your merits and demerits, that in Boston you were considered to be 'eccentric in dress'. Perhaps your cravat was included. Anyhow—*reform* before it is too late—." As an afterthought, he added: "For a man who dresses as I do I think the above is very good."[28]

The two hit it off. Besides his regular Washington visits, Dr. Chadwick voyaged frequently to Europe, always in the company of his *Want Book*, a thick leatherbound notebook with handles containing the Lib-

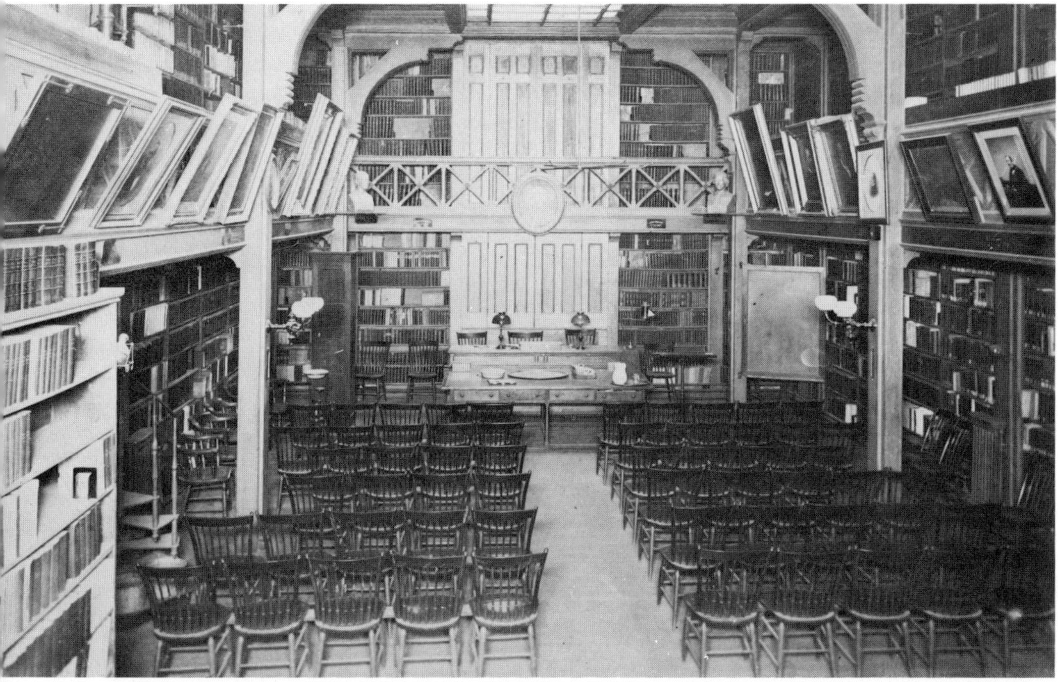

Meeting Hall, 19 Boylston Place, 1900

Reading Room, 19 Boylston Place, 1900. Dr. Brigham is seated. James F. Ballard stands at right.

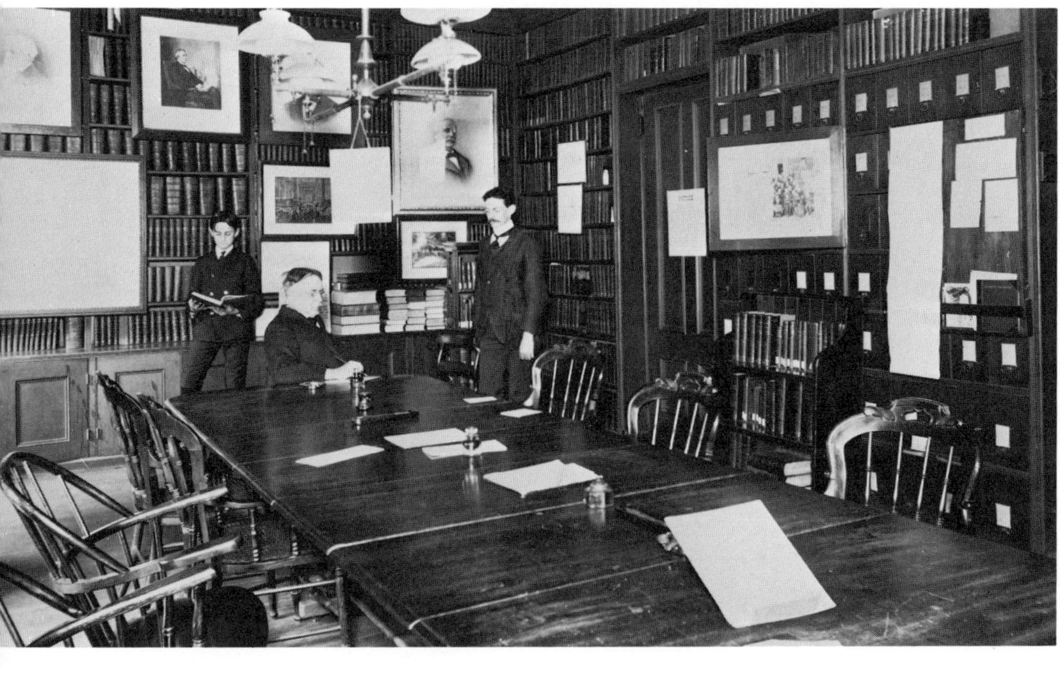

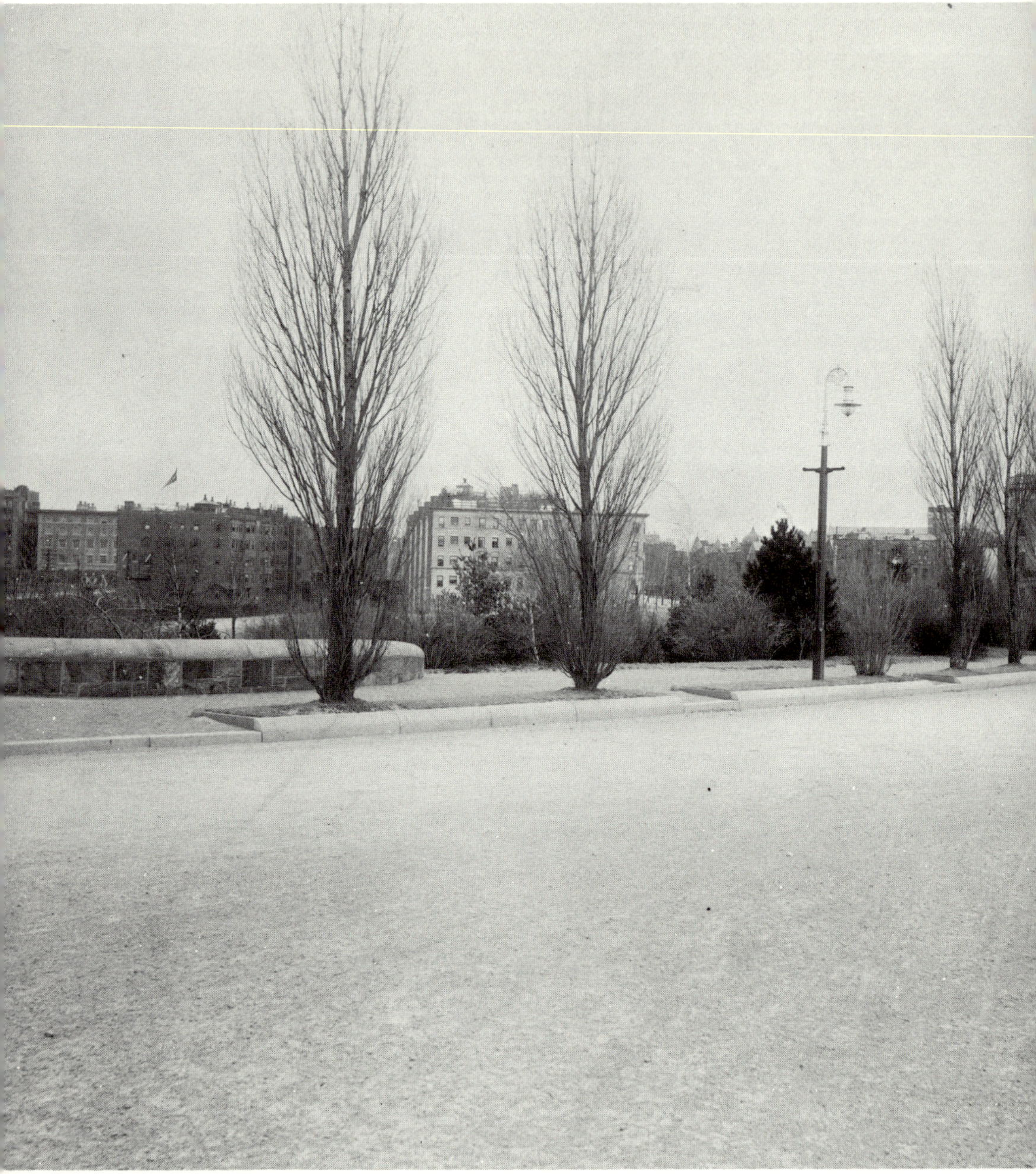

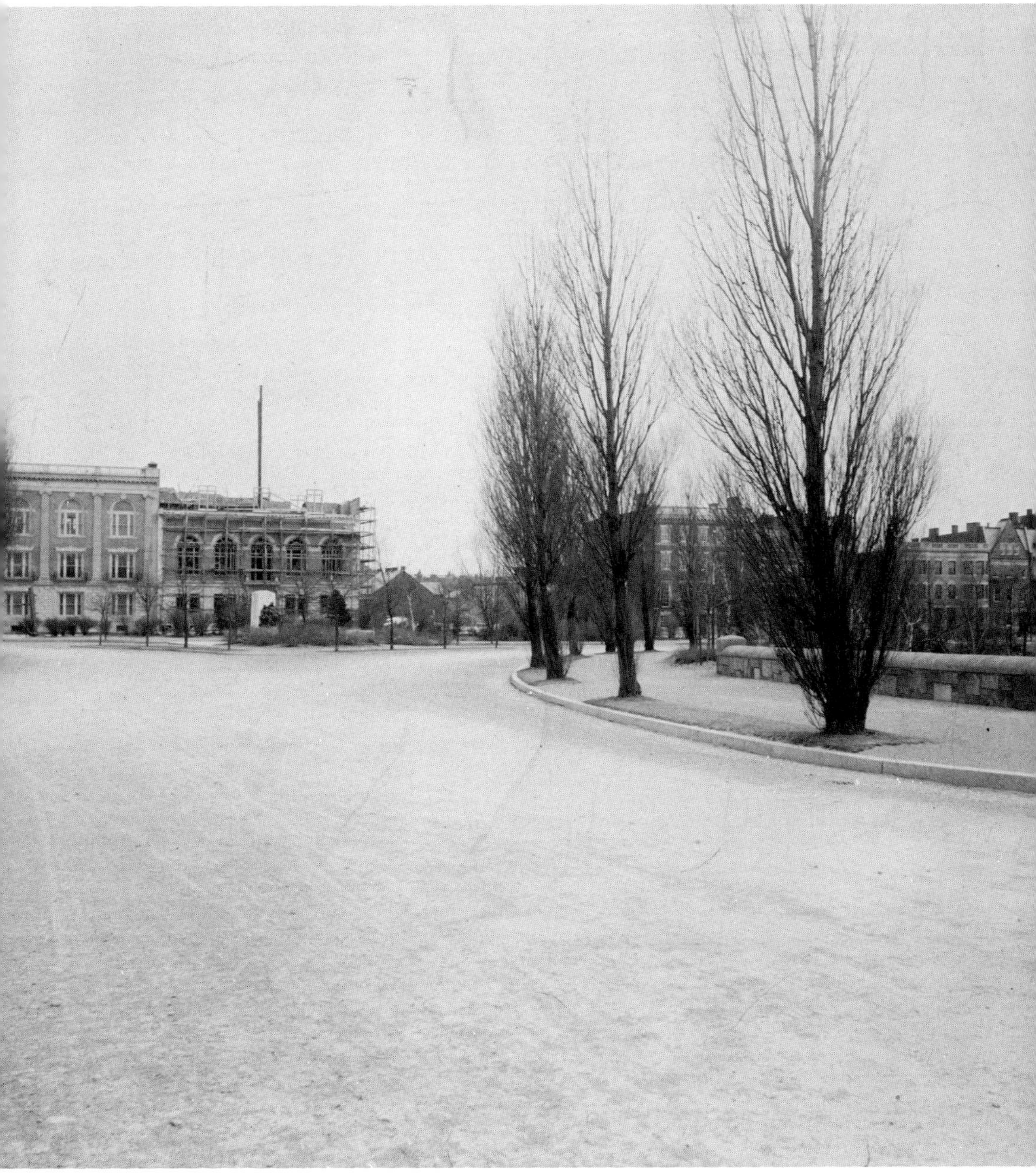

New library at 8 The Fenway under construction, probably 1900. The building of the Massachusetts Historical Society on the corner of Boylston Street at left was completed in 1899. Photo by the eminent Boston photographer Nathaniel L. Stebbins.

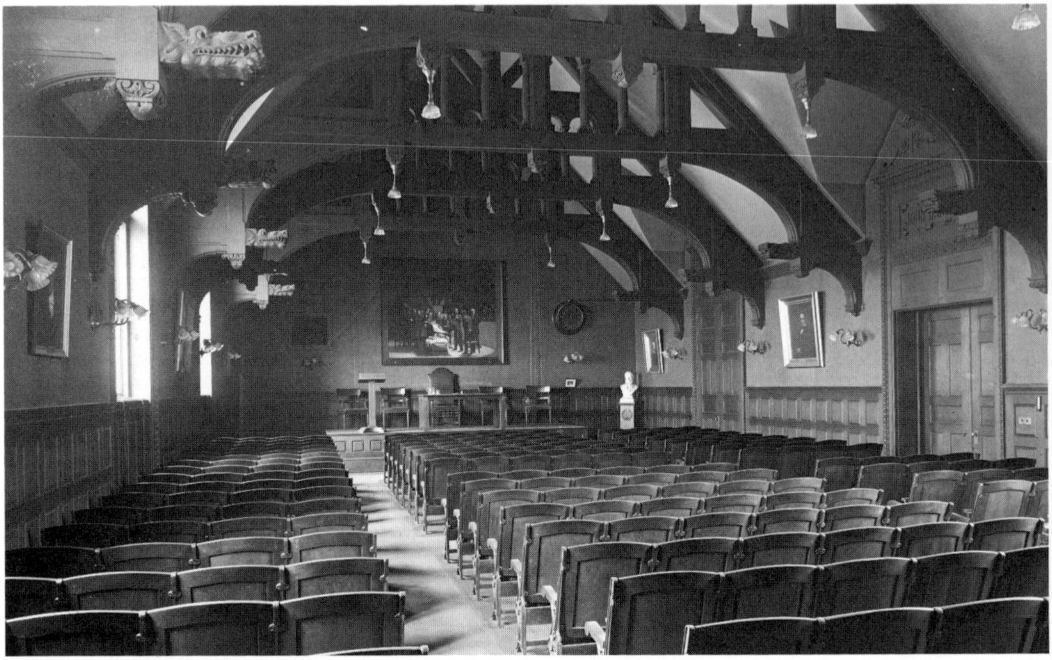

John Ware Hall, 8 The Fenway, 1918. The "Ether Picture" hangs on the far wall above the rostrum.

Holmes Hall, 8 The Fenway, 1918. Dr. David Humphreys Storer presides over the card catalogue at left.

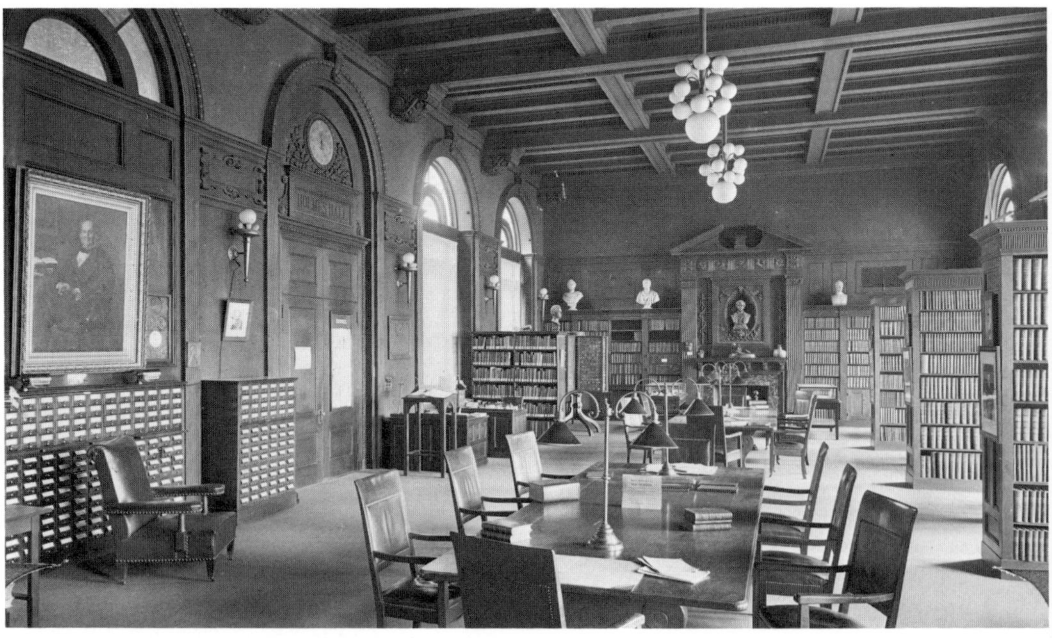

rary's "Periodical Deficiency List" painstakingly maintained to the minute of departure by Dr. Brigham in order that his superior might spring upon missing numbers of journals wherever they might lurk or try without avail to escape his roving eye in the capitals of Europe. He was a fearless hunter. On one safari to France he bagged hundreds of volumes he could not have captured by correspondence, as he explained, "owing to the indifference of the French second-hand dealers." At least once the two were travelling companions; following their return, Billings wrote Chadwick: "I want that game which we saw the Misses Longfellow playing on the voyage out—game invented by some Cambridge professor. Can the board for it be bought in Boston? Or can you tell me the number of squares on a side and get me a copy of the rules?"[29]

Goethe's *Ohne Hast aber ohne Rast* was Chadwick's *Grundsatz* and drove him ceaselessly in his practice, teaching, laboring into the night at the Library, corresponding, observing, writing, reading, fraternizing, lecturing, organizing the American Gynecological Society, championing the admission of women to Harvard Medical School and the Massachusetts Medical Society (Justin Winsor caricatured him at the end of a letter with the caption "This is the distinguished advocate of female medication"),[30] and cremation, of which he had the macabre distinction of being known as the *Father* in New England for his success at reorganizing in 1892 the New England Cremation Society, which the next year built the crematory and chapel at Forest Hills Cemetery.

The house which the Boston medical librarian created at 270 Clarendon Street, corner of Marlboro, after his return from Europe with his bride was singled out for imaginative description by an English travel writer, who found that since the filling of the Back Bay the new homes along Commonwealth Avenue had eclipsed Beacon Street:

> One of them, which impressed me greatly, is a noteworthy reproduction of an old English house. It belongs to Dr. J. R. Chadwick, a young medical man, who is rising to eminence in that important branch of his profession wherein the late Sir James Simpson excelled. If the earliest and greatest Governors of Massachusetts, Winthrop, Dudley and Endecott, were to enter this house, they would feel themselves more at home in Dr. Chadwick's dining room than in any other place in the city. They would tread a polished wooden floor, and see bay windows filled with lozenge-shaped panes of glass, such as were familiar to them in the comfortable homes of Old and New England. The spacious fireplace, in which wooden logs are laid across andirons, would recall to their memories many happy or thoughtful hours spent in youth or manhood beside the blazing hearth. The swords, shields, and helmets affixed to the wall above the fireplace would remind them of the weapons and armour which they had worthily wielded and worn. . . They would be able to sit, as they were wont to do, on high-backed Elizabethan chairs around the octagonal oak dining table. . . In the snug study they would observe other things to remind them of their olden

homes. . . I fear that the luxurious decorations and furniture of the drawing-rooms and bedrooms, though fashioned on Old English models, would seem to them far in excess of what sinful mortals ought to enjoy, and they might leave their excellent host and his charming wife with the conviction that it would be necessary to send the Rev. John Cotton to "deal" with them.[31]

His store of duplicates was his stock in trade. Dr. Chadwick cast this bread liberally upon the waters. Neither he nor his cause of *bibliotheca medica* could lose by his largesse. Digging into it, he helped to get more than one new medical library started on its way, as his friend Billings (in spite of his jest about that first "raid") had capitalized him with Washington cast-offs. As for what the tide might cast back, or when, he told of one such launching of loaves not long after the move to Boylston Place:

We have a library of 319 [*sic* 380] books which have a curious history. I sent a box or two of duplicates from our library to the University of Tokyo, and in return they sent me and my assistant, Dr. Brigham, each a handsome Japanese sword. They also said that a box of books had been sent us, but these were not heard from. Bunkio Matsuki, now of Boylston Street, had just come to Boston, and got the job of cataloguing some Japanese books at the Public Library. He reported that they were all medical books, and I found that the library people could not explain how they came into their possession. After something of a controversy, I made good our title to them [but not until 1887], and they were removed to Boylston Place. I paid Mr. Matsuki $40 for cataloguing them, which I understand was the first money he earned in this country.[32]

It was not simply that Chadwick was an acquisitor. As he pointed out in his 1886 report, the avalanche of literature produced by the divisions and subdivisions of the new science of medicine into the specialties was piling up directly at the doors of the profession, and its libraries, released in a sense by the agency of the Surgeon General's Library and the *Indices*. The cheerful warning of John Billings, *to him that hath shall be given*, was all too prophetic and only added to the congestion. Fifteen hundred volumes had been received from Harvard Medical School by the exchange agreement, another six hundred from the library of the late John O. Green, of Lowell. The volume census in only two years jumped from 14,799 to 17,124. Patronage was so brisk that the executive committee felt compelled to vote Dr. Brigham a dollar a week extra to be on hand Tuesday and Friday evenings. And on top of that, he must have an assistant, and Richard F. Daly was hired at four more a week. . . such a smart lad that in a year they were paying him six. Always recruiting, the Librarian drafted Dr. John Woodford Farlow (HMS 1877), a young laryngologist starting practice nearby on Clarendon Street, to give his spare time to helping Mrs. Collins with the catalogue.

Consequently, few members could have been surprised when Dr.

Chadwick broke the bad news in his 1886 report: the Howe house after only eight years was outgrown, and they must have an "absolutely fireproof building and accommodations commensurate with the value and size of your library. A new and capacious building in a less crowded locality is imperatively called for."[33] His call was heeded. In October of 1887 the Library bought for $15,000 a ten thousand foot lot at the corner of St. Botolph and Garrison streets.

Mrs. Holmes died after a lingering illness in February 1888. Without the support of his daughter Amelia, widow of Turner Sargent, who came to live with him in his Beacon Street house, the aged Autocrat could not have pulled himself together to touch his friends for several thousand dollars toward the price of the building lot in the months that followed, as he did.

His loss, and his age, bore heavily on Dr. Holmes. He had been thirteen years President of the Boston Medical Library, not onerously, but by holding on to this last of his professional associations he designated it, as Chadwick said, as the institution "in whose existence he takes the greatest pride, in whose future he has the greatest confidence."[34] Now, at seventy-nine, he felt he could no longer carry on even as the figurehead he had once protested he would never be, and in October of 1888 he passed the presidency to Dr. Richard Manning Hodges. It remained in the family, so to speak, for Dr. Hodges had started his brilliant surgical career as Holmes's demonstrator in anatomy and completed (after decades undeservedly in the shadow of Henry Jacob Bigelow) when age and deafness pushed him into retirement from the MGH in 1886.

Forsaking the obituary role of testimonial recipient, Oliver Wendell Holmes turned the tables on his old students and with that incomparable instinct for the *à propos* which had so charmed a large segment of western civilization presented his own medical library of 968 volumes to the institution which owed so much to his wisdom and example. It was the largest private collection yet received, and was formally accepted in ceremonies at Boylston Place on January 29, 1889.[35]

Dr. Chadwick expressed the pupillary feelings of the members toward the wizened old celebrity who had led most of them through their anatomy. "We elected Dr. Holmes president in 1875, when we formed this association, with the conviction that his name and his wise counsels would guide us over the perilous early years of the institution; and with the belief that if we should merit his approbation we should achieve success." Now, though junior among the seven medical libraries in the country, it ranked fourth with its nearly twenty thousand volumes. "This we feel is a very good showing; and we feel that the gift that we have received today of all these books of Dr. Holmes's is a proof that he is satisfied with the work that we have done."

It was a poignant moment for the Sage of Boston, enfeebled and depressed as he was, this hour of parting with the familiar stepping stones, as he called them, of his medical career which he had so carefully collected and saved over nearly sixty years, but he was up to it. The first acquisition he could remember, he told his hearers, was Bell's *Anatomy*, the oldest a copy of Avicenna printed in 1490 [and the nucleus of the Library's great collection of medical incunabula], the newest an 1887 text. Between the extremes of age "is a long, dreary interval, filled up by books not old enough to be curious or even rare, and not new enough to represent the existing state of knowedge." Yet they deserved better than contempt as "mere treasuries of unwisdom. The débris of broken systems and exploded dogmas form a great mound—a *Monte Testaccio* of the shards and remnants of old vessels which once held human beliefs. If you take the trouble to climb to the top of it you will widen your horizon; and in these days of specialized knowledge, your horizon is not likely to be any too wide."

The departing President spoke affectionately of his titles, "a formidable phalanx of grand old folios which give dignity to the lighter volumes beneath which they gravitate to the lower shelves," the odd, queer "rusty old volumes in this collection which will rarely, if ever, be taken from their shelves except to be spanked and dusted," his special loves, the anatomical works. . . the plates of Albinus, Vesalius, Mascagni's lymphatics, Soemmering's organs of sense, and the figures in the huge Spigelius which "will always attract attention, for the grace and beauty of the females who display their viscera as if they were their jewels and laces. These are not likely to be overlooked by the lovers of undisguised nature and naked truth."

And in parting:

> These books were very dear to me as they stood upon my shelves. A twig from some one of my nerves (as I remember saying long ago) ran to every one of them. From the time when I first opened Bell's *Anatomy* to that in which I closed my Sharpey and Quain and my Braithwaite's *Retrospect,* they marked the progress of my studies, and stood before me as the stepping-stones of my professional life. I am pleased that they can be kept together, at least for the present; and if any of them can be to others what many of them have been to me, I am glad to part with them, even though it costs me a little heartache to take leave of such old and beloved companions.

5

The Dignity of the Profession at Stake 1889 · 1901

Gay and free-wheeling the Nineties have survived in the popular mythology; in fact, the century departed the stage in tatters, hat in hand. Depression, panic, unemployment, strife and insecurity pursued the *fin de siècle* almost to its end. The times could not have been less favorable for shaking down the hundred thousand dollars required to fill the Boston Medical Library's vacant lot next to the Copley Square railroad yards with a well-ordered arrangement of bricks and books.

Only one serious moneyraising effort was mounted. It was in 1893. Frederick C. Shattuck had bowed off the executive committee and been replaced by John Homans 2nd, that dedicated demonstrator of the successful (that is, aseptic) ovariotomy who would have established abdominal surgery at the Massachusetts General Hospital thirteen years before its belated acceptance in 1889 had his true worth been recognized at the time of his appointment. Dr. Homans as usual was out front. He had plans drawn for a new building and got the rest of the executive committee to accept them and to make a stab, at least, at soliciting funds. But by September of 1893 the new building kitty had increased a pitiful $1500, to $10,000. The campaign was abandoned.

All the while, as if he had been cast as the sorcerer's apprentice in Dukas's frenzied scherzo, Jim Chadwick gripped his bewitched broom, and the more frantically he wielded it, the deeper the inpouring flood of accessions. There was the filling-in of the dental section on the initiative of the Harvard dental faculty, the enlargement of laryngology with the libraries of Franklin H. Hooper and Hamilton Osgood, the implantation of the Wigglesworth Library of Dermatology from the books of the faithful Edward Wigglesworth after his decease in 1896, the gift of a historical collection relating to the advent of ether anesthesia from Dr. J. Collins Warren. And still the book tide rose. In 1896, seventy years after they had absorbed the first Boston Medical Library, the trustees of the Athenaeum invited the second to take the cream of its medical books, about five hundred of them; in this way some of the original library came to rest on the shelves of its later namesake, thereby establishing, after the fact, a sort of genetic link.

The Society for Medical Improvement also chose 1896 to relinquish ownership of its eight hundred bound volumes of periodicals which had been on deposit since 1878. This enabled the Library to boast that it now owned everything within its walls, swelled to amorphous proportions by the overflow of books and portraits which gathered dust, unread and unadmired, in the storage rooms of Harvard Medical School and the Museum of Fine Arts, Dr. H. P. Bowditch's barn in Jamaica Plain, and even the Forest Hills crematory, where "they are safe against fire but unavailable for purposes of consultation," as Chadwick explained with delicacy.[1]

Dr. Brigham, who was not by nature a malcontent, seemed to regard himself as subhostler of an Augean stable in the American Athens:

> The building is in a district which is rapidly becoming a business section with its dirt and noise. A structure will soon arise to the height of eighty-five feet and within twenty feet of our rear windows. This will mean an absence of all sunlight and the burning of gas early in the afternoon and on cloudy days, also a close and stuffy atmosphere in summer.
>
> The books and periodicals are crowded on the shelves as far as possible in double rows, every wall space is covered with shelves completely full and the floor is now under contribution. The current periodicals on the shelves of the reading room are badly crowded and cannot be readily seen or found except by the library staff. Every addition to the library with its present contracted quarters is an embarrassment. There being no reception or workroom for books, pamphlets and periodicals, they are taken into the reading rooms and fill the tables and floors till they can be cared for, very largely increasing the labor of the library force. The hall is nearly all the time full of cases and piles of books awaiting attention, which are in the way, limit its use for meetings and annoy those who attend them. The use for meetings of the upper front room and the hall vastly increases the library work as any books not arranged or catalogued must be stuffed into nooks and corners for the time being and then overhauled again, entailing double labor and increasing the liability to mistakes. The bulk of the books being kept in the hall compels large numbers to be brought upstairs to the reading room for use and then carried back.
>
> The Index Medicus and Index Catalogue open up all our files of periodicals and with the crowded condition of our shelves and the necessary absence of a proper arrangement and classification makes it often very difficult to find many periodicals. All these disadvantageous circumstances impair the use of the library and make proper administration difficult. The hall is in many respects a bad place to keep the books, it is damp and books mould in the summer. The rain water pipes from the L roof pass through it and have often leaked and overflowed and many books have been damaged. [The Library's own roof was not the only source of run-off. In 1897 the executive committee considered lodging a protest with the Boston Library Society, only to be advised by counsel on June 3 that its neighbor "had acquired, through a continuous enjoyment of more than 20 years, the legal right to dispose of its rainwater through the premises of the Boston Medical

Library."] Early attendants at meetings often misplace books which for a long time are supposed to be lost till they turn up in unexpected places. Frequent sweeping makes the books very dirty and a great deal of dirt and dust comes in from the cellar, especially as all the ashes must be carried through the hall to the sidewalk.[2]

Fortunately for his employers, Dr. Brigham bore these travails with the *aequanimitas* so widely counseled by that occasional admired visitor, Sir William Osler. Not so his salary, which was as meagre as they could get away with. The assistant librarian was fairly constantly at the executive committee for raises over the years of his long tenure, and his bosses wedged him pretty hard, knowing as they did that the Library was his main dependence. His salary in 1890 was $1350. His boy Daly departed and was succeeded by Maximilian John, who by 1891 was exacting the imperial tribute of eight dollars a week. That was not far below the wages of Mrs. Collins, the assiduous and invaluable cataloguer, who received a well earned raise from twenty-five to thirty cents an hour in 1892. Maximilian held sway in the stacks until the fall of that year, when his place was taken, on October 24, to be exact about it, by a young fellow named James Francis Ballard, just turned fourteen by five days, who had landed in Boston from Saranac Lake, upstate New York, by way of Montreal, New Brunswick and a public school education which had terminated forever after a single month's experience of the eighth grade.

Ballard would make his mark on the Boston Medical Library, and on medical bibliography, but he was a green stripling now, in days not forgotten fifty years later by Henry U. Holzer, heir to his father's Bromfield Street bindery, U. Holzer, Inc.:

My first recollections of Boylston Place are very strong with me today. I have a very vivid feeling of the old place, the meeting room, which seemed to me an awesome cave; walls, stairs, landings, rooms, closets, all lined with books, and the heartening presence of Dr. Brigham, who was the most invigorating personality I have ever known. . .

In August, 1888, I carried my first load of books from Boylston Place to Bromfield Street, in a small wheelbarrow, inherited from my small-boy predecessor. The whole distance was paved with round cobble stones and to a small country boy's self-consciousness, even a small wheelbarrow can seem to fill the air with clatter, from Cambridge to South Boston.

It did not take long before I learned to transfer the laceration from my pride to my body, by carrying what the wheelbarrow would hold on my shoulder. By the time Mr. Ballard entered the service, transport was in the hands of my successor, who, being city-bred, was not bothered by the clatter of the wheelbarrow. It was therefore somewhat later that I made Mr. Ballard's acquaintance, and we became James and Henry, and began to travel down the years together.

Presently we were chartering a horse and team for deliveries and pickups, and by 1912 gasoline displaced oats for our transportation. I hope and trust that we may not have to revert to the wheelbarrow.[3]

Mrs. Amelia Holmes Sargent died unexpectedly in April 1889, hardly more than a year after she had picked up stakes to keep house for her grieving father in the wake of her mother's death. She left the Library $25,000, payable on the passing of her father and her brother, Justice Oliver Wendell Holmes of the Massachusetts Supreme Judicial Court, who, with his wife, succeeded her in moving in to care for his father. The Library would not become beneficiary for another forty-six years.

Dr. Holmes died on October 7, 1894. He was eighty-five. The executive committee reacted emotionally; it met immediately, summoned a special memorial meeting of the Association for October 30 and voted to recommend to the members that the name be changed to "The Oliver Wendell Holmes Library." However, second thoughts prevailed. On the 30th the committee modified its recommendation—that the principal hall of the new library when it was built be called "Holmes Hall." The name was adopted at the memorial convocation later in the day.

Dr. Francis Minot had succeeded Dr. Hodges as President in 1890 and was in the chair. He recalled that he was one of Dr. Holmes's first pupils in the proprietory Tremont Street Medical School, supplementary to Harvard's around the windy corner of Mason Street. Former students, now eminent, gave vent to their memories, affectionately, amusingly, trenchantly, of their venerated Professor. . . Thomas Dwight, C. B. Porter, Henry Pickering Bowditch, George B. Shattuck, editor of the *Boston Medical and Surgical Journal* which published the proceedings[4]. . . these and their fellows joined in recording their "admiration of those qualities of mind and heart which made him the most eminent and best beloved member of our profession in America."

His portrait, painted by E. T. Billings in 1889 when Holmes retired as President, was presented to the Library by Dr. Clarence J. Blake on behalf of the subscribers, to be hung in Holmes Hall when there was one. Blake related how diffident the subject had been about sitting, and what difficulty he had persuading him, mainly on the strength of the artist's recent rendering of Henry Ingersoll Bowditch, which Holmes viewed at Blake's home before its presentation to the Library and considered a good likeness and thought "he had never seen Dr. Bowditch quite so spruce before."[5] Yet the famous subject remained skeptical, and the first two sittings did not bode well. Billings asked his wife to drop into the studio casually for the third and sit with the sitter. Blake read from the notes Mrs. Billings jotted down afterwards:

> The third sitting was a remarkable one. Dr. Holmes said there was a good foundation. He stood before the picture and talked on the anatomy of his face, and went over all the muscles, giving their names. He was delighted to learn that

Mr. Billings had studied art anatomy with Dr. Rimmer, and that he was receptive and sympathetic on this subject. His faith grew, and that helped the work wonderfully. He became more at ease; was playful, witty, beaming; and at the close of this sitting studied the painting, and said, "Well, Mr. Billings, you have got the old man. You have the *equilateral* under the nose, made by the middle of the upper lip, the lower part of the nose, the full muscle of the cheek and the upper lip. No one gets that. You have it; and without it there can be no likeness of me—hereafter—for expression". . . When finished, he was enthusiastic in his commendation of the portrait, and added, "You have made me look like a gentleman; the coat is a credit to the tailor."

To Blake: "Yes, it is there; the age is there; the wrinkles are there. It is a likeness. It is the portrait of an old man; dew-lap and all." And not long before his death: "The portrait grows upon me. I think that it is the likeness of me that will stand."

Which is not to say that age could ever entirely extinguish those final faint flickers of the Holmesian vanity. At the memorial meeting Chadwick displayed a bronze of the autocratic fist by the sculptor Truman Howe Bartlett, and told how "Mr. Bartlett as he was about to cast the hand, asked Dr. Holmes if he would hold a pen. He said, 'No; take it that way (the fist closed tightly); that does not show the old man's wrinkles, does it?' "[6]

The members abbreviated the Boston Medical Library Association to the more permanent-sounding "Boston Medical Library" on March 13, 1896. Dr. Francis Minot this year was seventy-five and stepped aside for his vice president, David Williams Cheever, another of Dr. Holmes's "boys" by dint of having followed Richard Hodges as his anatomy demonstrator thirty-five years back. In 1893 Dr. Cheever had retired as Professor of Surgery at Harvard, where he was to be long remembered as a lecturer of lucidity and precision. At City Hospital he was a visiting surgeon from its founding and continued as president of the staff. He was a former president of the American Surgical Association and the Massachusetts Medical Society. Now he was sixty-five, tall, somewhat stooped, so spare as to give the appearance of frailty, but of Puritan steel to the core. Whether on the podium or at the bedside, in the operating room or in the larger theater where he fought many a public health battle (*an unflinching leader,* J. Collins Warren called him), Cheever painstakingly prepared his ground and then moved forward with decision, imagination, and often considerable boldness. Harvard recognized his sagacity and influence by welcoming him as an overseer this same year of his elevation to the presidency of the adolescent library which Dr. Brigham in his 1896 report likened to "the young man coming of age. . . strong and lusty, continually outgrowing its clothes until now they are full to bursting."

Dr. Cheever's ascendance coincided with what by 1898 had taken hold as an unmistakable improvement in the economy, and with the entry into practice of Frederick J. Cotton (HMS 1894) and Elliott P. Joslin (HMS 1895), one in surgery, the other in internal medicine with whisperings of interest in diabetes, neither yet thirty. Co-conspirators, these two were, in "a band of the younger men who felt strongly the hindrance to their studies and researches by the fact that the resources of the Library were not available [and] started an agitation which the governing board of the Library welcomed and fostered."[7] So wrote the Librarian approvingly.

Their tub-thumping resulted in a special meeting on November 29 at which Dr. Cheever pronounced 19 Boylston Place "not worthy of the dignity of the regular profession in this community" and declared it unthinkable that remedial funds should not be forthcoming.[9] Chadwick asserted that "the diploma of M.D. merely certifies that its possessor has laid the foundation of the knowledge essential to enable him to combat disease and death; upon the superstructure he must labor to the end of his days. . . A library is consequently indispensable in every centre of population, or the health and lives of the community will be jeopardized by the ignorance of its medical practitioners." Invited by Cheever to speak for the younger members, Cotton stroked any feathers which may have been ruffled by their agitation; he contented himself with an invidious comparison of reference facilities in Vienna to the *efficiency* of Dr. Brigham's operation, which must have brought a blush to that good man's cheek.

Dr. Coll Warren, staunch advocate of the best in medical education, exhorted his young colleagues that if they would step forward and do their share, "the stones of the new building would pile up upon one another in no time at all." He foresaw the Library giving the physician the opportunity to be always the student in its primary role as an institute of postgraduate education, indeed, as evolving in its new quarters into a gathering place for the profession akin in aim, scope and atmosphere to the College of Physicians in Philadelphia and the New York Academy of Medicine.

All fired up, the members pledged to raise $100,000 behind the lead of Dr. Cheever. The matter of the location of the new library, however, was left to an ad hoc committee of J. B. Ayer, Arthur H. Nichols and Walter L. Burrage. Distaste for the lot at St. Botolph and Garrison streets had been growing; it was central, but the region of the railroad yards was diminishing in dignity by the day.

The agitations of Cotton, Joslin and their crowd resulted, in the hyperbole of the Librarian, in "the uprising of the whole medical profession of Boston and its suburbs,"[9] and the tree which sprouted from the seed gift of $20,000 from an anonymous lady friend of the Library soon was shedding its green.

The three-member committee on site, meanwhile, had debated itself into a state of fractional impotence, judging from their report that they were *evenly divided* between the admittedly unattractive building lot already in hand, and two (and possibly three) in the wide open bush of the recently created Fenway which they had been inspecting, next on the south side to the new headquarters of the Massachusetts Historical Society under construction at the corner of Boylston Street. Along here, from Jamaica Pond to the Charles River, the westward-pushing frontier of the Back Bay fill in the eighties had bogged down in the *Stygian morass*, as Walter Muir Whitehill describes it, of the foul and fecal flats of the Muddy River until the landscaping genius of Frederick Law Olmstead converted it brilliantly into the almost hygienic and adaptable park known as the Fens.[10]

The deadlocked three reported in its favor that the Fenway location would appreciate in value, that it had a tolerable rear and an unsurpassed front view, that in short it was "quiet, clean, bleak"—as it certainly was, for it was virgin made land (anomalous but true). They added without much enthusiasm, in the words of President Cheever (whom they asked to summarize their dilemma and to call a special meeting to resolve it, if possible):

> It is objected that this place is not central—never will have around it the population, as it gives on a park and a river; that it is not accessible; that the doctors to the east and southeast, Roxbury, Dorchester, etc., strongly oppose it; that it is no place for a Nurses' Bureau; that it is bleak and unhandy for seven months in the year, and that it will remain so. The nearest electrics are on Massachusetts Avenue and Ipswich Street,
>
> In rebuttal it is said that this site is the only one worthy of the dignity of the profession, and that a handsome building there will bring us notice, money, and reputation.[11]

The argument at the special meeting on May 25, 1899 was hot, because Dr. Joslin brought in the proxy vote of Dr. Grace Wolcott which made a tie and stopped the St. Botolph-Garrison street proponents in or near their tracks. Then, by fifty-three to nineteen, the members voted to sell 19 Boylston Place (it went to Joseph Walker, for $23,500) and to buy the pair of Fenway lots to build on for $24,000, and the adjacent third to the south, against the future, for $18,000. Thirty-two thousand dollars was reported as having already been subscribed. To sweeten the Fenway pill, Joslin and Cotton pledged that the young Turks would guarantee the interest on $25,000 for five years at four per cent.[12]

While the Boston Medical Library was coming to grips with its future, Harvard Medical School—quite as full to bursting a few blocks away on Boylston Street—agonized in a quandary over its. During his deanship a decade earlier, Henry Pickering Bowditch had found what he imagined as the answer to the need for nearby clinical facilities under the School's control, à la Hopkins, in the will of Mr. Peter Bent Brigham, a wealthy Bostonian who died in 1877 and left behind a trust to build a hospital for the sick poor of his city, but not before 1902. The date was approaching. The trust had swollen to over five million. With predatory intent, Dr. Bowditch tried to persuade the faculty on June 3, 1899—a week after the Medical Library had decided on its move—to recommend to the University that land be acquired for a new school and hospital. He was rejected.

Possibly the Library's fundraising success, the excitement generated by the sight and sounds of the edifice designed by Shaw and Hunnewell rising on the bank of the Fens under the guidance of the building committee (J. C. Warren, Farrar Cobb and Chadwick), and not least, the halving of their apartness by the move, helped to activate the medical faculty; on May 5, 1900 it cast hesitation aside, changed its stance and voted to urge that the twenty-six-acre estate of the late Ebenezer Francis along Longwood Avenue, once the shore of the original Back Bay, be acquired for a new school with the understanding that it be acceptable to the trustees of the Brigham will as the location for their hospital. Dr. Warren preferred a magnificent tract on the Boston side of the Charles closer to the University, now the site of the Harvard Business School,[13] but he downed his reservations and consented to be chairman of this building committee also, with Dr. Cobb as consultant. Thus were interlocked the grand designs of School and Library.

The Francis estate was remembered by that small son of the bookbinder, Henry Holzer, rattling his wheelbarrow over the cobbles:

> In the earliest days my godparents occupied a cottage on Longwood Avenue, exactly where the Richardson House of the B. L.-I. now stands. For a coincidence, Dr. Richardson was the first human to set eyes on me.
>
> Opposite the cottage, from Longwood Avenue to Francis Street and from Huntington Avenue to Vila Street, was an apple orchard, and where the Peter Bent now stands I have played three-o-cat. I suppose Peter at that time was in full cry after the dollars with which to transform that land.
>
> Behind the cottage, as far as Massachusetts Avenue, was only marsh and creek, where we children skated and ran teets when I visited on winter days. Not one of the great assembly of institutions now there existed except in dreams.[14]

With the closing of the century the Boston Medical Library deserted "that diverticulum of hidden dangers, that Bohemian midway pleasance," as Dr. F. W. Draper described Boylston Place, for the bleak bank of the meandering Muddy River. After ninety-five years of packing, unpacking and repacking from private homes to apothecaries, from Athenaeum to Public Library, from rented rooms to a barn and a crematorium, the medical literature of Boston had come to rest on shelves worthy of its dignity. The move to 8 The Fenway cost about $140,000 when the bills were in, of which $73,000 was collected by Dr. Homans's subscription committee, including five hundred from the Harvard Medical Alumni Association which Chadwick had founded at a meeting in the old place on November 26, 1890. After sale of the diverticulum, a $50,000 mortgage remained as a reminder that the twentieth century would probably not be all pleasance. The Librarian sought counsel from Dr. Billings, now at the head of his most recent creation, the New York Public Library, who advised him how to arrange his periodicals in the new layout, "putting the Homeopathic, popular, etc., in the most distant part of the stack in alphabetical order,"[15] a rustication which would have pleased Dr. Holmes.

The facade of 8 The Fenway (the building was party-walled against the Massachusetts Historical Society) was a sombre brick upon granite. The entrance was surmounted by a decorative balcony. The great arched windows were imposing underneath a row of dentils and three finialed dormers. More or less Romanesque, and very quietly so. Dignified.

The visitor possessed of the weight and strength to grapple open the ponderous front doors found himself in an octagonal hall of choices which might lead to the Nurses' Directory, the Supper Room (for the use of the Massachusetts Medical Society) and the Smoking Room. If one penetrated the corridor straight ahead, one passed the staircase and elevator well (liftless for lack of funds) and came upon a small meeting room in the rear, Sprague Hall, panelled and columned in dark oak, ceiled in moulded plaster, furnished and hung with portraits in memory of Dr. Richard Sprague (HMS 1887) with a gift of $5000 from his brother, Congressman C. F. Sprague, and their mother.

The climb to the second floor led to the periodical and catalogue rooms and the first level of stacks which were intended to hold 50,000 books and failed miserably of the mark. These were the heart of the Library, but its soul was in the main reading room, Holmes Hall, seventy-two by thirty-two feet, splendid in its oak and flooded with light from the expansive windows which overlooked Mr. Olmstead's landscape, sombre in its fine carved wainscoting and Norman timbered ceiling, learned in its stands of well-weighted Greek revival bookcases, each presided over by one of the familiar busts, those *lares et penates* lugged up from Boylston Place, stern and admonitory with its long tables set so stolidly upon their clawed feet and the chairs upholstered in leather thick enough for a minimum of comfort and thin enough to insure a maximum of productive application.

A surprise Holmes Hall bonus for those whose interests lay in that direction was the gift in 1900 from Dr. Horatio R. Storer of Newport, Rhode Island, of 2139 medals having to do with medicine which he had been twenty-two years in the gathering. Dr. Storer presented what was said to be the largest collection of medical numismatics in existence in memory of his father, Dr. David Humphreys Storer, with the stipulation that it be displayed (as it was, on swinging leaves) and that the old gentleman's portrait, which the Library had owned since 1889, be hung nearby. His son, Dr. Malcolm Storer, was to be curator.

Dr. Chadwick suspended the forceful but kindly visage of the senior Storer above the card catalogue, midway between the portrait of Dr. Holmes by Billings and his bust by R. E. Brooks, which gazed at each other, as if their subject were smiling inwardly at himself, from the ends of his Hall. Here were noble shrines to that medical man of letters without rival, matching marble fireplaces under mantels and panels of glowing oak, consummately carved, framed within twin columns rising from the hearthside to support the lofty broken pediments that crowned the whole creation, olympian, oracular, inspiring, worthy of the autocrat, and of the profession which doubly glorified that small and humorous man. Beneath his graven images were his books, his revolving study bookcase, his two old easy chairs, his bronze clenched fist, a doorlatch from the place of his birth. . . it was as if he had arranged it all himself. . .

> I love sweet features; I will own
> That I should like myself
> To see my portrait on a wall,
> Or bust upon a shelf;
> But nature sometimes makes one up
> Of such sad odds and ends,
> It really might be quite as well
> Hushed up among one's friends![16]

Although Holmes Hall occupied two stories from floor to ceiling, the remainder of the third was called the intermediate floor and contained behind the stacks, as if in quarantine, a chamber originally designated the Students Room (the students soon were driven out by the inflow of reading material) and a smaller meeting place, the Fifield Room, furnished in memory of Dr. William Cranch Bond Fifield of Dorchester (HMS 1851) by his widow.[17]

Above Holmes Hall, under the ridge of the main roof, was the auditorium, seating three hundred. It was unfinished when it served for the dedication ceremonies, and then during 1901 Dr. and Mrs. Charles M. Green came forward with $5000 to furnish it as a memorial to Mrs. Green's father, Dr. John Ware, one of the eminent proprietors of the first Boston Medical Library. Dr. Ware died a few weeks after his son was killed in the Civil War in 1864, inspiring Dr. Holmes to write "In Memory of John and Robert Ware," soon after his agonizing search of the battlefields for his own wounded son:

> These blood-red summers ripen fast;
> The sons are older than the sires;
> Ere yet the tree to earth is cast,
> The sapling falls before the blast;
> Life's ashes keep their covered fires,—
> Its flame expires.

Ware Hall, when complete, was the Valhalla of the Fenway. The Greens' gift touched off another run on dark oak, so that the inside perimeter could be lined with wainscoting, leaving still enough trees in the forest to mill and carve with the heaviest of hands into perfectly massive trussed rafters which were hoisted up and secured in some way as if they were supporting the high, vaulted cathedral ceiling. But this was no cathedral, more a feudal manor hall or the feasting place of dour deities of the north, for each great, incredibly ugly timber was seemingly trunnelled to the wall by the hidden body of an awful dragon whose head glared across the void at its identical adversary, its pupils dilated, its mandibles bared, its molars at the ready, its nares all but aflame.

At the rear-alley end of the third floor a largish room was reserved for meetings, but soon it too was suffocated by books. Almost needless to say, there was no room at the top for an assistant librarian's apartment. As much had been made plain to Dr. Brigham during the planning, and in 1898 the executive committee had consented to his removal from Boylston Place, as he had requested, on the condition that he accept a salary cut sufficient to hire a replacement during his off hours. A year later the committee rather curtly informed him it was not aware of having promised him an allowance, as he seemed to think it had, on account of rent in lieu of an apartment in the new building.

The Boston Medical Library's home on the Fens—President Cheever's "chaste and appropriate edifice"—was dedicated on January 12, 1901.[18]

The founding Librarian was perhaps not altogether in earnest in suggesting that the day was at hand for "we men of '75. . . we silverites" to give way to the next generation. James Read Chadwick was fifty-six. It was his day, and there to help him celebrate it, as he had been twenty-two years earlier in a similarly outrageous meeting hall, was John Shaw Billings, who was now running his most recent creation, the New York Public Library:

As you all know, these results are largely due to the fact that one man having abundance of energy and public spirit, with much knowledge and an insatiable thirst for more, and with a fairly definite idea of what he wanted, has been working incessantly for the last quarter of a century towards this end. I congratulate you upon your wisdom in letting him thus work, and in helping him to carry out this plan. His power for good has not been limited to Boston, for by way of recreation he has devoted some of his time to stirring up and stimulating other librarians like myself, when he thought they needed it, or when he had some superfluous energy to dispose of, which was often. In this and other ways, he has given material and valuable assistance to other libraries, more than any of you are aware of, and it is not my personal affection for him, great as that is, but a sense of what is just and right, which leads me to say to you that, while the Boston Medical Library has been his special pet, for which no trouble was too great to take, and no sacrifice too great to make, all other medical libraries in this country are more or less indebted for their progress and prosperity to your librarian, Dr. James R. Chadwick.

Dr. William Osler, who owed his professorship of medicine at Johns Hopkins to Billings, was present and added his own assessment, and some words of Oslerian wisdom:

The feeling which absorbs all others is one of deep satisfaction that our friend, Dr. Chadwick, has at last seen fulfilled the desire of his eyes. To few is given the tenacity of will which enables a man to pursue a cherished purpose through a quarter of a century—"*Ohne Hast, aber ohne Rast*" ('tis his favorite quotation); to fewer still is the fruition granted. Too often the reaper is not the sower. Too often the fate of those who labor at some object for the public good is to see their work pass into other hands, and to have others get the credit for enterprises which they have initiated and made possible. It has not been so with our friend, and it intensifies a thousandfold the pleasure of this occasion to feel the fitness, in every way, of the felicitations which have been offered to him. . .

Books have been my delight these thirty years, and from them I have received incalculable benefits. To study the phenomena of disease without books is to sail an uncharted sea, while to study books without patients is not to go to sea at all. . .

Osler expressed his special affection for the book-lovers, the "bibliomaniacs. . . the leaven of the whole lump," and he wanted more of them, especially in America,

where every one carries in his pocket the tape-measure of utility. Along two lines their work is valuable. By the historical method alone can many problems in medicine be approached profitably. . . But in a more excellent way these

> *laudatores temporis acti* render a royal service. For each one of us today, as in Plato's time, there is a higher as well as a lower education. The very marrow and fatness of books may not suffice to save a man from becoming a poor, mean-spirited devil, without a spark of fine professional feeling, and without a thought above the sordid issues of the day. The men I speak of keep alive in us an interest in the great men of the past and not alone in their works, which they cherish, but in their lives, which they emulate.

Dr. Cheever agreed:

> From the walls of Holmes Hall, from other rooms, look down upon us the portraits of many of our medical forefathers and teachers: The Warrens, Bigelows, Jacksons, Homans, Shattucks, Wymans, Bowditches, Cabots, Putnams, Storer, Ellis, Buckingham, Holmes! How can I cease the enumeration? These were scholarly doctors. We need to continue this patrician *Gens*. Science enlightens, but does not wholly satisfy; the humanities in education soften manners, nor allow them to be harsh. The moral effect produced on the patient and the community by the learned, as well as gentlemanly, physician, is great and wholesome. Let the doctor cultivate books, and let the influence of this library help him to do so.

It was left to Dr. Chadwick to take the measure of the day, and of the first quarter century of his Library:

> We knew [in 1875] that the era of theories and systems in medicine was being pulverized into nothingness by the accumulation of crude facts and that these facts were to be found chiefly in periodical literature. Periodicals were then increasing at so rapid a rate that few private individuals could afford to obtain, or even give, them shelf room. We did not at that time foresee that this difficulty was to be increased a hundredfold. . . by the publication of a colossal index [the Index Catalogue] to all previous medical literature, including every article in every one of the numerous periodicals. . . Its value to medical scholars is inestimable, superseding, as it does, all the time-wasting labor that used to be expended on bibliographical research. By its aid we obtain a reference to every rare case that has been recorded since printing was discovered in A.D. 1450. But by indexing the articles and reports of cases in every periodical, past and present, obscure and famous, this catalogue has immensely extended the scope of medical research and created a demand for an array of books, and especially of periodicals, that is simply appalling.

In an earlier circular letter to the profession, President Cheever had announced that the privileges of the new library would be extended beyond Boston throughout Massachusetts. . . that "this is to be an Academy of Medicine, a Medical Club, and meeting place, and the future home of the Massachusetts Medical Society."[19] And on this day of dedication the *Boston Globe* noted that the Library "no longer discriminates against women, and about 20 are now members and permitted to avail themselves of the privileges of the place." Dr. Chadwick approached the subject of the future only slightly less unequivocally than did Dr. Cheever, wondering if "now that we have secured the library and the best equipped building in the country in which to store it, we may properly consider whether the time has not come to enlarge the scope of our functions by assuming the role of a society in addition to that of a library." Recalling the authority with which the College of Physicians of Philadelphia advised the government in the quarantining of a yellow fever epidemic many years earlier, in contrast with the absence of such a body of medical men in Boston, he imagined its counterpart in his home city, moving forward and outward from the cultural and scientific base of the Library to embrace the "philosophic brethren" of the medical profession in a more inclusive instrument for the exercise of social responsibility and public health leadership.

It was not by chance that Dr. Horatio C. Wood, the noted Professor of Nervous Diseases and Therapeutics at the University of Pennsylvania, sent greetings from the College of Physicians and devoted his address (*in absentia* at the last minute) to a discourse on its merits and an admonition to Boston to go and do likewise.

The day, and the century, closed with a message, grave and graceful, from Dr. S. Weir Mitchell, enjoying at seventy-one (though not immoderately) the fullness of his fame as the Holmes of Philadelphia:

Philadelphia, December 29, 1900.

Nothing, my dear Chadwick, except engagements, not to be broken, keeps me from being among those who in person congratulate the profession on the opening of your new library. To you more than to any other I send my gratulations, for to this end you have given costly days out of a busy life.

I see as I grow old, or may I say older, how few are the young medical men whose tastes are scholarly, and who, like Holmes and our lamented Da Costa, are familiar with the fathers and find pleasure in the old books—the quaint books, the sense and the vagaries of the past. Without a great library few can afford these intellectual playgrounds, or, indeed, acquire the material for such indulgence.

May your new building and growing wealth of books tempt many into paths where some of us have found unlooked for treasuries of interest and even of practical value; for indeed the dying century did not invent common sense, and genius is of every age.

I often remember with regret the great waste of time in my younger days when there were no great libraries, and when John Billings had not indexed the medical thought of all the centuries. The enormous labor then in any mere literary research as to facts no one can imagine today. A great library of medicine is truly a labor-saving machine, and over your library and over its new home you should rejoice because a great library, well managed, practically lengthens life by saving time.

My thin thread of New England blood seems to be tingling with friendly pride as I reflect on what the profession has here accomplished. I send you my greeting from the city I love best to that I love next best, and wish you all, and the newly instituted library, long, useful and honored days.

As I pause to assure you how truly I am yours I am conscious that I really have more and better things to say; but as like as not others will have said them, and I leave therefore to the eloquence of suggestive imagination all the fine things which I am tempted to say and will not.

Believe me, my dear Chadwick, always and in all ways,

Your friend,

S. Weir Mitchell[20]

The uneasy promise of the infant century which confronted the Boston Medical Library on this day of its maturity was delivered in wry benediction by its godfather, John Shaw Billings:

The collection of books, of portraits, of medals, the building in its plan, structure and furnishings, are all things of which you have good right to be proud, and with which you may rest satisfied for several weeks to come.

6

Flood in the Fenway

1901 · 1918

Build thee more stately mansions, O my soul,
 As the swift seasons roll!
 Leave thy low-vaulted past!
Let each new temple, nobler than the last,
Shut thee from heaven with a dome more vast,
 Till thou at length art free,
Leaving thine outgrown shell by life's unresting sea!
The Chambered Nautilus

All the while the foundations were being laid for the newest temple on the Fenway, Dr. Holmes's unresting sea (the poem begs the analogy) so flowed as to cause Librarian Chadwick to warn uneasily that its completion "will give us another high tide, which will deposit upon our shelves books in number far in excess of any flood that we have seen in the past,"[1] a spring tide released from the reservoirs of the barn in Jamaica Plain and the crematory in Forest Hills, and swollen with the dammed-up collections whose owners and guardians awaited only the vaulting of a vaster, and fireproof, dome to shut them in.

The waters rose faster than ever Chadwick had expected, though small relief *he* provided by bailing aboard (while he was sure there was room for it) his own catalogued library of 3000 pamphlets and 500 to 1000 volumes (he was vague as to the total) dealing with his specialty, mostly. The inundation filled much if not most of the basement of the new building from floor to ceiling. Chadwick got two or three volunteers to help him at the pumps, chiefly Dr. Farlow:

> Dr. Chadwick was equal to the task and laid out a plan which was carried to completion. He worked at it several hours nearly every day including Sundays and holidays, and sometimes also in the evening. Being Chairman of the Library Committee, I was pressed into the service, unable to resist his goodnatured invitation to help the good work along. I have seen him drop in on his way to a dinner party, in evening dress, and do half an hour's work, so as to hurry up some particular task that he was anxious to finish.[2]

The job took two years and produced as a by-product a duplicate library of 3000 volumes, 101 cases of additional surplus that were given to sixteen medical libraries around the country as needed, and a bonanza for the scrap paper man. The sentimental casualty was the Librarian's treasured Want Book, which after going through three editions in manuscript had finally to be shelved itself by the impossibility of keeping it up to date.

The next wave left 3700 castaways from the Harvard College Library's medical section, consisting of the old Boylston Library and the Jeffries books whose inaccessibility across the Charles led to the founding of the first Boston Medical Library. The College Librarian, W. C. Lane, offered them on deposit in June 1902 and congratulated himself in his annual report that he had thereby gained "a little free space. . . I think there is no possibility that we shall ever want to recall those that relate to purely medical subjects."[3] Most were of historical interest only, and about half were duplicated at the BML.

The third tidal wave to lap the filling stacks at 8 The Fenway (an affectation of address, by the way, presumably intended to set *this* Fenway apart from all imitators, as *The* Country Club in Brookline) had been activated a quarter of a century in the past by the patient Chadwick, when he tried to wheedle from Dr. Morrill Wyman his most prized literary possession. Bowditch's collaborator mentioned the attempted raid on November 1, 1878: "You once asked me for the deposit of my Tiedemann Library. I was obliged to decline because it is the only medical library in Cambridge to which I have access; if I lived in Boston you should have it."[4] Chadwick persisted. . . there was "probably no other collection in this country so complete up to the publications of the middle of the last century."[5] Wyman had acquired these 3987 volumes and 4125 pamphlets of plates and classics in anatomy, physiology, zoology and early medicine from the estate of Friedrich Tiedemann, Professor of Anatomy and Physiology at Heidelberg. After the move to Boylston Place Chadwick tried again. This time Wyman deferred until fireproof quarters were available; but then he changed his mind, tired of waiting, and gave everything to the new Cambridge Public Library. He died on January 30, 1903. In December the Cambridge library trustees eagerly offered the Tiedemann collection to Chadwick on deposit, and were relieved when he as eagerly accepted all 212 boxes.[6]

The move to the Back Bay had established the Boston Medical Library with the hard-pushed general librarians as the welcome repository for the medical literature in the area, which accounted for the fourth wave of the flood. The Boston Public Library had hurdled the BML to Copley Square in 1895, only to be outdone at the game in 1901, and now sent word of its willingness to make of 8 The Fenway a deposit station for such of its 10,000 medical books, plus serials, as the doctors might select, on the condition that their ownership be identified and they be accessible to the cardholding public. The first of the pick drifted down Boylston Street in 1906; a decade later 11,000 had beached out above the Fens before the ebb set.[7]

Chadwick's predicted tide bore more than books. In May 1903 the trustees of the estate of Robert Charles Billings gave the BML $50,000, of which a fifth was to be reserved as a permanent income fund in his memory for book purchases, the balance to be thrown against debts, namely the mortgage. No one seems to have been exactly sure who Mr. Billings was, but the executive committee felt as grateful as Harvard did in 1900 when his trustees bestowed $93,610 on the new Medical School.

The Billings bounty was followed in 1904 by Mrs. Sarah E. Potter's bequest of $150,000 to erect, complete or enlarge a building as a memorial to her late husband, on the straightforward condition that it be signified the "Warren B. Potter Memorial" by a bronze tablet over the entrance. The building had arisen in the meantime, but this seemed a small favor in exchange for such a legacy, especially since Mrs. Potter's will permitted the Library to use it for furnishings or maintenance as it chose. The tablet was attached to the balcony, looking rather an enigmatic afterthought, and in three years the money was received with interest, $159,000. Mr. Potter had been a partner with Andrew J. Weeks in the Boston drug firm of Weeks and Potter. George Robert White, another benefactor of Boston, started with them as a boy and cleaned up as the Cuticura soap king, controlling owner of the Potter Drug and Chemical Corporation, one of the largest wholesalers in the country.

With an arthritic foot uncomfortably in each century, the old and crusty Society for Medical Improvement assembled in annual meeting on January 21, 1901 in the fine new Fenway home of its stepchild, nine days after the dedication. Dr. Edward H. Bradford, about to occupy (in 1903) the first fully upholstered chair of orthopedic surgery at Harvard, presided and posed a question which remains unanswered: "None of us know whether this century is to be an iconoclastic one or not, whether it is to look upon the work of the nineteenth century as an entertaining diversion simply, or whether it is to respect and draw inspiration from the recent past."[8]

Those few present who expressed themselves agreed that *their* Society, in any event, was in a state approaching the moribund which Dr.

James C. White, who was about to vacate the first chair in dermatology at Harvard, attributed to too many medical associations, all competing for the practitioner's time. This palpable view of the case was followed by the pathological findings of Dr. Reginald H. Fitz:

> Those of us who recall to mind the Medical Improvement Society of thirty years ago realize that a marked and undesirable change has taken place in its spirit. The society was established for the improvement of its members at a time when medical progress was slow and medical centres were widely separated, if not in distance, certainly in the interchange of ideas. The relatively few members who had enjoyed superior advantages in the acquisition of knowledge and experience were called upon to advise and assist the less fortunate. The meetings were largely attended by the leaders of the profession. . .
>
> In the meantime a revolution has taken place in medical progress and a retrocession in the importance of the society. . . As specialty after specialty became represented in the membership a growing number of communications of interest to the few only were presented. Attendance at regular meetings thus was limited to an increasing minority of members subject to constant change in its composition. . . Now we are led to the thought that the Boston Society for Medical Improvement may have outgrown its usefulness and should retire in a dignified manner before evidences of decay become painfully apparent.
>
> We must remember, however, that all physicians are not specialists, that the leaders in the medical specialties are those whose training in medicine has been the broadest, and that the ideal association of physicians in communities of sufficient size is that which includes the representative men of each and all departments of medicine. Any association which can bring these together and hold them together always is needed.[9]

Dr. Fitz picked up Dr. Chadwick's call of the previous week for a Boston Academy of Medicine with the blunt suggestion that it be conceived of a union of the Improvement Society and the Medical Library, "since the aspirations of the latter may trench upon the functions of the former." Library open to all, membership "to those only whose association would prove mutually beneficial". . . subjects of general rather than special interest for presentation and discussion, meetings social as well as medical, celebrated guest speakers on live topics. . . these measures, Fitz thought, should restore the purpose of the Improvement Society "to improve the knowledge, power and influence of its members."

The first of a succession of study committees was appointed, while the Library sounded out the social side of the equation with a sequence of nonscientific smoke talks beginning in June with Dr. C. J. Blake's reminiscences, striking a high in December with a talk by William Osler on Thomas Linacre and concluding, without a trace of the iconoclasm suspected by Dr. Bradford, in May of 1902 with steropticon views and anecdotes of the old-time surgeons by Dr. George H. Monks. Encouraged, the Improvement Society that spring joined with the BML in a committee to pursue the academy will-o'-the-wisp under Dr. William T. Councilman, the breezy Hopkinsian who had succeeded to the chair of pathological anatomy when Fitz moved over to the Hersey professorship in 1892, thereby becoming the first "outsider" to occupy a front-row seat in the history of Harvard Medical School. The initial assignment of the Councilman committee was to plan six wide-ranging clinical symposia for the coming season, for the sake of which the Improvement Society declared a one-year moratorium on its own ill-attended scientific gatherings.

The academy test was decidedly positive in the presence of such reagents as Councilman expounding on the skin lesions of variola, Bradford on congenital dislocation of the hip, Painter on bone tuberculosis, Joslin on urea assay and his classmate Harvey Cushing and the latter's friend from Cleveland, George W. Crile, on the unusual notion that there might be advantages to monitoring blood pressure on the operating table. The meetings were a revelation to the Improvement Society's subcommittee, chaired by the surgeon James G. Mumford, which that winter prepared a draft blueprint for an "Academy of Medicine for Greater Boston" and published it as banns for the affianced in March of 1903.[10] The year happened to be the Society's hundredth. Mumford had written of its rise and decline and had been committed to the academy scheme for over a year.[11] Viets considered him "somewhat of a medical reformer, although not of the aggressive, disagreeable type."[12]

The Mumford committee picked up where Fitz left off. It agreed that in its early days the Improvement Society fulfilled the function of the contemporary special club by taking in the best men in the local profession when they were few and the science of medicine could be encompassed by a single bright intellect. But by continuing to admit only the best it had grown too large for uniformity of purpose, yet not enough to meet the demands of a general society; it was regarded with jealousy and suspicion by many of the younger men and exercised scant influence on public opinion. Quite simply, the old Society had had its day.

On the other hand, in the committee's view, a dominant factor in the success of the meetings at the Boston Medical Library was their democracy. The democratic idea was the key to the success of the general society, and to whatever immortality the Improvement Society might hope to aspire. Therefore, "we propose to expand it only, by combining it with the permanent and indestructible Library; for we believe that only by giving a clinical society a habitat and large vested interests, such as the Library carries, can it be made permanent. If so combined, the clinical interests of the Society might die or might change indefinitely in character, but with its large property and increasingly great membership, the organization of which it forms a part could never come to an end."

The Mumford committee suggested that the Academy draw its membership from within ten miles of the State House, that it maintain a medical library, conduct medical meetings, run a directory for nurses and "consider all medical questions affecting the public; i.e. hygiene, sanitation, etc." The BML, according to its plan, would apply to the state Commissioner of Corporations for permission to enlarge its functions and revise its constitution accordingly, whereupon the Society would vote to unite with it and apply to the court to be allowed to give up the corporate ghost.

All this was a swan song more proud than pathetic, when one considers that 180 of the 193 active members of the Society belonged to the BML, whose predecessor it had hatched ninety-eight years back, and amounted to nearly half of the Library's roll of 388.

With the publicizing of these recommendations, events moved rapidly to a resolution, though not the one anticipated. Within weeks a slightly modified plan was adopted, first by the executive committee of the Library and then by the Society, which on June 1 voted to transfer its assets to the Academy, when and if created, and to suspend scientific meetings. Twelve days later a special meeting of the Library directed the clerk to apply to the Commissioner of Corporations for authority to change its name to "Boston Medical Library and Academy of Medicine" and to expand its purpose. And then came the hitch: the Commissioner advised that the unanimous vote of every member was required. This was patently impossible, and the annual meeting in November instructed the executive committee to ask the legislature to change the charter.

Its dying act delayed by these unexpected changes in the scenario, the Improvement Society a trifle deflatedly rejected the Library's invitation to finance a second series of clinical meetings for the 1903-1904 season and decided to resume its own.[13] The BML's discouraged executive committee pondered the implications of a change in charter and gave in to second thoughts itself. To be an effective voice in medical matters, it was argued, the Academy would have to be more selective in its admissions than the Library (certainly contrary to the Mumford committee's expectations), which would have the effect of reducing income precisely when the contrary was called for.

In January of 1904, three years after it had been conceived with the more-than-willing Medical Improvement Society, the officers of the Boston Medical Library aborted the Academy of Medicine and chose an alternate means to the same general end of broader membership participation, education and influence: new by-laws. These were adopted by the corporation that May. Henceforth the president would be elected by the members, no longer by the executive committee from its own. There would be three vice presidents in place of one, with overlapping terms. The executive committee itself was eliminated as the governing body in favor of a committee on library and finances consisting of the officers and five members; with the new committees on medical and social meetings, and on membership and elections, it formed the council of the corporation. Four classes of membership were created: Fellows (formerly active) paying the new dues rate increased from eight to ten dollars a year; associates (added on moving to the Fenway), paying five; life; and honorary.

The appeal of the Academy persisted. The Medical Library arranged a revival of the clinical meetings with the Suffolk District Medical Society and in October issued a membership broadside: "The object is to unite in one body the best members of the profession of Greater Boston; and, as far as possible, the whole State. This will be an 'Academy of Medicine.' "[14]

A nearly forgotten remembrance remains, pasted inside the cover of every worthy orphan volume acquired by the Library. In an overflow of wishful thinking, Dr. Chadwick had hired an artist to draft a bookplate, *Academia Bostoniensis Medicinae*, with the motto *Servat et Docet* above a wreathed representation of the semi-clad Aesculapius seated by a tree, an oriental plane, perhaps, around whose trunk clung the healing serpent; against it in a relaxed pose leaned a gentlelady, probably one of the god's health-giving daughters, Hygeia or Panacea; at their feet a ram received the ministrations of a boy, doubtless the therapeutic prodigy, Telesphorus. Twin torches kept the light aloft above the scroll *Fundata MDCCCLXXV*. When the Academy came to naught, the Librarian scratched out *ACADEMIA* for *BIBLIOTHECA*, had the design engraved, and so it remains as the bookplate of the Boston Medical Library.

L. S. Ipsen, the artist, also designed a circular seal for the BML in English except for the motto, which was spread across an open book between two torches. An element of the inspiration behind these emblems may be traced to the learning which the first president wore so lightly:

296 Beacon St. Jan. 29th [no year]

Dear Dr Chadwick,

I looked [in] my little book which was *not* "Alciati Emblemata" [*Emblems*, by Andrea Alciati (1492-1550)] but "Idea Principi Christiani politici" of Saavedra [*Empresas politicas, o idea de un principe politico cristiano*, by Diego de Saavedra Fajardo (1584-1648)] without finding anything peculiarly appropriate. Alciatus (or ti) is common and worth looking over—you can find it in any of our public libraries.

I return your two figures—one, rather—but not the pens which are wonderful and if I had not my gold pen in a quill as you drew I should be envious of you and perhaps hire a professional to steal them from you.

An open book with a torch and the legend *Lucet, Ducit, Salvat* might be thought of, but no doubt you can find one worth a dozen of it.

Yours very truly

O. W. Holmes

A heap of letters to answer—so excuse haste.[15]

The bookplate and the seal were among the last and least of James Read Chadwick's contributions to the Boston Medical Library.

He was found dead outside his summer residence at Chocorua, N.H., on the morning of September 23, 1905. On going to bed the previous evening he appeared to be in his usual health. It is supposed that he was taken ill during the night and went to the dangerous narrow balcony outside his bed-room in the second story for air, stumbled and fell over the low railing to the ground below, striking on a Japanese stone ornament in his descent, as attested by bruises found on his head and side. In his hands were portions of the vines which he had clutched as he fell. The medical examiner gave it as his opinion that death was accidental and was due to abdominal hemorrhage caused by the fall.[16]

Dr. Chadwick was sixty. At the annual meeting of the Library on November 14 Dr. Clarence J. Blake, who had put his shoulder with him to the founding of it, took the measure of his old friend:

. . . Of James Read Chadwick it may be said that his personality, as exhibited in his relations with his human kind, was an effective part of the equipment by means of which he achieved that which he undertook and also, that its effectiveness was a basis of the persistence with which he followed any undertaking for good. . .

Essentially a medievalist in his tastes, with a strong sense of the joy of living and an equally strong joy in the labor of accomplishment, as strikingly individual in his habit of dress, the picture of him as we call it to mind, is that of a cavalier, or of a knight errant on single quest, whose mission was rather to succor, to comfort and to uplift, than to fight and vanquish. . .

His sense of humor, his lightheartedness, his raillery were the silken shoulder-cloak beneath which he wore his shirt of mail flexible, and but hardly penetrable. On ground that he believed, or pretended to believe, to be firm, he was no mean controversialist and the blade of his wit hung, not in a clinging scabbard, but in a hip knot, and was quick in lunge and ready in recover; in the very mien and carriage of him, on such occasions, there was that which runs between the lines of one of his favorite later poets, "The sweet sound of steel upon steel in the joyous passage of arms at Ashby."

If the dress, simple but unconventional, set forth the man, so also did his chosen surroundings, the office in which he received his patients, alone, never, though thereto urged, in the presence of an office nurse, because, as he said, his patients were entitled to a privileged communication—seemed quite as much a library or a museum as an office; the spaces between the windows, and the walls, where not hung with sketches, portraits, and curios, were covered with books; the single table heaped with manuscripts and letters, from which complex mass, after due stirring, any desired communication, recognized by a protruding corner, would be seized, withdrawn and submitted to perusal. . .

It was a place in which to sit cozily of an evening, between lamplight and firelight, with comrades, or with the silent companionship of books and writing work, as the late glow of his windows often testified, and the very furniture of the room bespoke its hospitality, the chairs were so easy to slip into and so very hard to get out of. . .

Of the professional work done in that office, the personal testimonials are many, not merely work in his especial line of service, but in the broader sociological field which is the opportunity of every physician. "I never," said a good woman whose daily life carried her much among the needy of her sex, "took a poor girl to Dr. Chadwick that he did not give to her his personal attention and to help me in what I had to do for her". . .

His responsive versatility enabled him, while pivoted upon his own centre of thought, to turn quickly to any magnetic point upon the horizon, like the needle of a compass, or to swerve toward it, like the versatile anther of a flower, and did much toward the making of those varied friendships which he enjoyed, and through which he sought to serve, and which were all instinct on his part, with a happiness in being helpful. Through this combination of versatility and constancy he was led to ignore the lesser qualities in his new found friends and to point straightly at that which made for distinction. . .

To his collaborators, and especially to young men and young women, entering the medical profession, he was most generous of his time, of his judgment, and of more material help. . . The very last occasion of his visit to Chocorua, where he met his death, was the freeing from difficulty of a patient, and the provision for her maintenance during the remainder of her life. After an evening passed in working with his lawyer toward the fulfilment of this purpose, he said, "Now that is done, let us have some music and go to bed," and so went to his rest and was seen alive no more. . .

To us, with the memory of him so immediate, portrayal is not needed, but it is good to have the assurance, for those who come after, that his portrait will find its place here. So strong, so clear, so instinct with his life, is this our immediate memory, that it seems almost as if that door should open and that he should enter, that we, assembled in this building, the embodiment of his keen desire, should be as indeed in verity we are, his guests, and he the genial, hospitable, welcoming host.[17]

They named the periodical room after him and elected John Woodford Farlow his successor.

Dr. Farlows's association with the Library went back to his student days in the class of 1877 at Harvard Medical School. He trod the usual postgraduate route through the European medical centers, and on regaining Boston entered laryngology, for a specialty was all the rage in those days for the bright young Americans. In 1895 he invented the widely adopted Farlow punch and the Farlow snare. In seven more years he was president of the American Laryngological Association. He was Clinical Instructor in Laryngology at Harvard, on the staffs of City Hospital and the Dispensary, fifty-two years of age, an old friend and neighbor of his predecessor, and he had been chairman of the library subcommittee of the committee on library and finance since the reorganization of 1904, after ten years on the executive committee. Dr. Farlow's credentials, then, were impeccable. He was a dignified gentleman of New England Puritan caste, dry-humored, cultivated, a first-rate pianist, and if not the compulsive prime mover and collector Chadwick was, a knowledgable connoisseur of medical literature and no less devoted to the Library.

November 1906 marked the seventy-fifth birthday of Dr. Cheever and the completion of ten years as president divided between Boylston Place and the Fenway, a ripe time to step down for George Brune Shattuck, the genial editor of the *Boston Medical and Surgical Journal.* Dr. Shattuck was sixty-two, handsome and arresting behind his parted beard, grandson of George Cheyne Shattuck the senior and elder brother of Frederick Cheever, diffident concerning practice and teaching, though fully conscious of the responsibilities attached to his family name which elevated him to Harvard's Board of Overseers and the presidency of the Massachusetts Charitable Eye and Ear Infirmary. His main interest since 1881 had been the *Journal*, to which he brought literary grace and wit.

The guard was indeed changing.

Dr. Brigham was sixty-nine in 1909, and not well, and retired as assistant librarian. With his ready graciousness, always behind a good cause, Dr. J. Collins Warren raised a $10,000 trust for this faithful and unprepossessing man whose salary, as Dr. Warren said, "has scarcely sufficed for the support of his family and has permitted no accumulation for his advancing years."[18] After the deaths of the Brighams, the principal was to become the Edwin Howard Brigham Book Fund.

The place of the Civil War private who had leaped from a clerkship to Harvard Medical School without stepping upon a single stone of higher education was filled by that same James F. Ballard whom Dr. Brigham had hired for his lowly stack and errand boy fourteen years earlier, at the age of fourteen. The new assistant librarian had shown such capacity for self-education and had so well versed himself in library technique under the guiding hand of Dr. Chadwick, who shaped his quickness in the periodical direction, as to make himself indispensable to the Librarian's successor, who must have elevated "James" with relief as he found himself at once trying to stare down the throats of his patients and cope with the inundation which had swamped this stately mansion of which he was the caretaker. In 1911 Dr. Brigham was appointed Library Curator, and Ballard's salary was raised from $100 to $150 a month provided he give full time to the job, which implies that the enterprising chap had more than one iron in the fire.

Illness and age caught up, too, with Oliver F. Wadsworth, the meticulous secretary since the very beginning, later clerk as well, and in May 1911 he resigned. On November 29 Dr. Wadsworth died, in his seventy-fourth year. "Nothing in his life became him better," wrote Dr. Shattuck, "or deserves our imitation more than his manner of leaving it. He went almost directly from the golf links to the operating table, and though the verdict was against him—meaning months of discomfort, of pain, of weariness—there was from that time no complaint and no flinching from the inevitable. . . Above all, he was a resolute, an honorable and kindly gentleman."[19]

The Library did not have far to look for its second secretary. While practising gynecology, Dr. Walter L. Burrage (HMS 1888) had served on the executive committee from 1896 and on that three-man panel which reported itself "equally divided" over the choice of a new site in 1899, and he had been in the forefront of the campaign for an Academy of Medicine. In July of 1903 he was stricken with poliomyelitis and lost the use of his legs. Forced into a sedentary life style, he turned to writing and other desk pursuits such as the secretaryship of the Massachusetts Medical Society in 1909, and now like service for its landlord.

At the end of his first year Dr. Farlow felt compelled to call to the attention of the members in his 1906 report that accessions were coming in so thick "we shall soon have to cast about for more shelf room, as we have already nearly reached our limit." A year later, in his 1907 accounting: "It is a very short, but a very sad story when we come to consider the condition of the stacks: they are full to overflowing, and some of the pamphlets will have to be transferred from the upper stories to a room in the basement to make room for our regular accessions." In 1908 three cellar rooms were fitted with shelves, and filled, "and we are again forced to cast about for more space."

A rumor in 1903 that the adjoining vacant lot was about to be bought up for a residence had prompted the Library to acquire it for $24,000. Six years later the basement of a future stack building was excavated and roofed over on it between the BML and the town house of the architect, Robert S. Peabody, for $5600. In twelve months Farlow was dismayed: "We had great hopes that this addition, capable of holding 30,000 volumes, would be all that we needed for several years; but I have now to tell you that this addition is already nearly full, and there are several thousand volumes still waiting to be transferred from our stacks and the crowded workrooms in the basement." A year later: "A new and very much larger stack-room is urgently needed in the near future."[20]

"It is all in-come and but very little out-go," the Librarian lamented to the annual meeting in 1912, "and we are seriously embarrassed for lack of space." This time he struck a spark in Dr. Morton Prince, that psychologist of fertile mentality who had but recently retired as Professor of Neurology at Tufts. Toward the end of the year Prince convinced the committee on library and finance that it ought to go after $75,000 to extend the basement stack foundation back to the rear alley and as high as it legally could, for 200,000 books. Too late. The effort evaporated into the First World War with only about $10,000 in hand, and this was invested in a stack of Liberty Bonds for the duration.

The invasion of books and journals did not slacken until half of Europe was in flames. Farlow's dirge for 1913 added even the Library's kitchen to the once off-limits areas which were now overrun, while "the periodical room has been practically only an encumbered passageway for two years. . . the floor is strewn with express packages. . . and both sides of the hall leading from the room to Holmes Hall are lined with piles of journals. . . the large hall in the rear of the upper story is so crowded with books that it is a sort of obstacle race to get through."[21] By 1915 the weight of stored tomes had oppressed the rear floor of the basement into the primordial muck of the Muddy River flats so alarmingly that it was necessary to remove them (where?) and shore it up with steel beams tied to the foundations and embedded in concrete.

The success of the Boston Medical Library in satisfying its clientele of course stimulated the expectations put upon its resources, and in true cyclical fashion the acquisitive prowess of those in charge who, aghast and yet elated over all that "in-come," measured their success since the pigeonhole days of Hamilton Place by the number of outgrown shells left behind on the trail. And still the tide rose.

Measured as items catalogued and not counting the hoard which was pushing the cellar floor out of sight (that is, estimating a mile with a yardstick), Chadwick began it all in 1876 with 121 journals in his current file. By 1913, the last year of peace, the BML had on hand 675 live periodicals. Translated into volumes, of which a great number were bound but by no means all, this represents a tidal wave, bounteous to suffocation, mounting a scale from 4488 to 78,080, not including the pre-war duplicate library of 7079. As for pamphlets, mean low water was first recorded at 5678 in 1881; in 1913 the wavelets lapped at 56,051. And then there were the 30,000 or so foreign theses which Dr. Farlow purchased in 1911 "at a moderate price" in Leipzig.

Not the deluge, certainly not, but the finite capacity of the reservoir was bemoaned. It had become a kind of a game, a bender, an orgy of collecting. After wading through the auctions and book markets of America and Europe, Dr. Farlow prayed for rain:

> There is a great mass of material relating to medicine which never comes into the market at all, but which could fill a very important place. Every physician has in his possession pamphlets, newspaper clippings, photographs of medical men, medical schools and buildings, biographical notes, autographs, etc., which are either soon thrown away or become destroyed by improper care. Numbers of out of the way journals are consigned to the junk dealer as old paper without a thought that they may be just what is wanted to fill a gap in a set at the library. It is better to send all such miscellaneous material to the library and let the librarian be the judge of what is of value. . . [Another point] is the advisability of the doctor's giving to the library during his life the books and journals which he wishes to contribute rather than deciding to leave them after his death.[22]

The heavens obliged. Farlow and his gasping staff flailed about upon a sea of private libraries, good, worthless and indifferent. . . and junk of every description. Specialty collections rained down. There was the excellent, continuing accumulation of the medical papers of his forebears given by Dr. J. Collins Warren and the section on diabetes added to over the years by Dr. Joslin. All was duly recorded in the annual reports, and borne on the back of the tide there was enough flotsam and jetsam to dampen the most ardent beachcomber—a pair of bellows, the advertising exchanges of Mellin's Food Company, a tanned human skin from the Tewksbury Almshouse, a pouch made from the epidermis of a pirate hanged on Boston Common, and a volume of the memoirs (perforce in limited edition) of the highwayman George Walton, bound in his own hide.[23]

This quintessential predicament of the dynamic library—forever trying to stuff hundred-pound lots of paper into fifty-pound bags—laid upon the BML the compounded burden of gleaning from a periodical literature which dwarfed the afflictions of the custodians of the other special fields of knowledge, not to mention all but the most inclusive general libraries. Within its purview the problem was as wide as it was deep. The perimeter was expanding rapidly under the influence of the new science. *Biology* was no longer merely a cover for botany and zoology, as Farlow was discovering. "Mental science," as he called it, and psychology were knocking for admission, joined by a diverse crowd of applicants, all claiming interest. . . tropical medicine and veterinary, bacteriology, biochemistry and the other burgeoning basic sciences, even that tenuously applied twig of a graft, called, for short, phys ed. . . and unthinkable of the unimaginable, "the various forms of faith cure, Christian Science, mental healing and psychotherapy, have compelled the librarian to add works on these subjects to his already crowded shelves."[24]

Furthermore, by consenting to be the Public Library's deposit station for medical literature, the BML had acknowledged its responsibility as virtually the exclusive home of the region's, which Dr. Farlow was rather ahead of his time in observing "is assuming a much more extensive relation to the community at large than ever before and is less restricted to practitioners of medicine. This fact imposes on the Medical Library the duty of opening its rooms, under certain restrictions, to the general, non-medical public; it means a much greater use of its books, a much larger interest in its success and consequently a more important position in the educational world."[25]

Attendance records, first kept with care in 1904-1905, confirm Farlow's observation and prediction. During those twelve months there were 3103 member visits and 3497 by non-members. By 1913, the pre-war benchmark, member registration had not increased to speak of; it was 3340. But there were 9291 visits by non-members. It is of some interest that Dr. Chadwick embarked on these seas with 133 cohorts; they were 365 in 1899, on the eve of the move to Muddy River, when the roster swelled to 672 in 1906, and 699 in 1913, of whom 474 were Fellows, 214 associates, ten life and one honorary. William Osler was the first of the last category, elected in 1911. John Shaw Billings joined him in 1912, died in 1913 and was replaced by S. Weir Mitchell, who died in 1914, leaving Sir William once again alone on the summit.

Most of the visiting non-members had been Harvard medical students. In 1897 these limited privileges were extended to Tufts. In the same year, however, "complaint having been made that the library rooms were so much used by students that members were practically excluded," these minors in the family of medicine were banished from Boylston Place except during the morning hours.[26]

Harvard's free-loading was irksome. On December 26, 1900 the executive committee asked the medical faculty to come across with some financial help, pointing out that the new building would be much more useful to the students, who had been enjoying the Library for nothing, and more costly to operate. It found an ally at the dedication a fortnight later in the person of Henry P. Walcott, M.D., Harvard's acting president, who expressed his outrage over the "absolute poverty" of the Medical School library's 2240 volumes, the skimpiest in the University. "The explanation of this seeming lack of care on the part of the university for her Medical School, in which she takes a just pride," he declared, "is undoubtedly to be found in the fact that the resources of this library have been most freely given to the teachers and students of the school. The authorities of the university may well consider whether some equitable arrangement may not be possible for giving to the library an equivalent for the valuable and necessary assistance so freely and generously bestowed."[27]

After a month, on February 9, 1901, the executive committee and its high-placed protagonist got their answer from the secretary of the medical faculty: it was regretfully not within the power of the School's administrative board to recommend an appropriation toward the maintenance of the Boston Medical Library. "Personal care for the students of the School," Harrington observed in his *History* published just as the marble-bound quadrangle of Eben Francis's old estate was about to be occupied in 1905, "had never been an object of much concern to the Medical Faculty."[28] During the planning of the new School the committee on university education in medicine suggested there should be dormitories, a dining hall and other facilities for students, including a reading room and a library. However, the concept of bibliographic home rule won out. "The idea of having departmental libraries," in the words of Dr. J. C. Warren (who with H. P. Bowditch raised the Morgan, Rockefeller and Huntington money that built the School), "was looked upon by the laboratory scientists as a distinct advance and much better adapted for quick reference than one central library. Experience seems to have shown, however, that under this system the student may not be tempted to use the library as freely as when a central locality encourages him to avail himself of its facilities."[29]

Conscience did prevail in the end, and after the Medical Library had been well settled in its new mansion the Harvard and Tufts faculties came through with $200 a year each. The poverty of the Harvard library which appalled Dr. Walcott also appalled Archibald Cary Coolidge, the historian who had been dedicating his spare time to uplifting the University's to "great" status, but he proposed quite a different cure. Coolidge had been appointed the first Director of the University Library in 1910. On April 15, 1912 Harry Elkins Widener, college class of 1907 and a keen booklover and a very wealthy one, went down with the *SS*

Titanic in the North Atlantic after seeing his mother aboard a lifeboat. By early 1913 Mrs. Widener and Professor Coolidge were discussing her desire to commit a portion of the family fortune to a university library in memory of her son. On April 11, 1913 Dr. Farlow recorded in his *Medical Library Notes* that Coolidge had proposed to him a merger of the Harvard Medical School library and the Boston Medical Library.

Ten days passed, spanning the first anniversary of Widener's death, and on April 21 the committee on library and finance received a formal proposal from Coolidge that the two institutions combine in a single library in the immediate neighborhood of the School, "with the object of obviating duplication of effort and making the Harvard Medical School the focus in this community of medical literature as well as of medical education." President Shattuck, Librarian Farlow and Secretary Burrage were constituted a committee to confer with Dean Bradford, Chairman Joslin of the HMS committee on library and Professor Coolidge. Farlow sounded out Dr. Fitz and found him "much opposed" to a merger.[30]

Delegated a one-man subcommittee, the Librarian of the BML reported on January 19, 1914 that "as, apparently, the Harvard Medical School has nothing to offer to the Medical Library, the sub-committee will devote itself to preserving most friendly relations with the Medical School and will endeavor to avoid in future unnecessary duplication in the purchase by the Library and the Medical School of the same books."[31] His view prevailed with the officers, who concluded, as Dr. Burrage phrased it in his 1914 report, that "no close affiliation seemed to be feasible without sacrificing the independence of the Library."

Professor Coolidge had one arrow left in his quiver, whether retaliatory is hard to say. In February 1915 he wrote the BML requesting the return of the medical books which College Librarian W. C. Lane had deposited there in 1902. Consultations were held with Dr. Farlow. Lane's disavowal in his 1901-1902 report of any interest in their return was produced, and the matter dropped. Coolidge had grander objects on his mind: the Harry Elkins Widener Memorial Library was formally opened on June 24.

Dr. Fitz's opposition to the Coolidge overtures was a final act of loyalty to the Library of which he had been a founder, an incorporator, a member of the admissions committee for twenty-two years and vice president since 1912. He died on September 30, 1913. He was seventy. President Shattuck spoke of him at the annual meeting in November:

> No one has made greater or more fruitful use of its resources than he. From the years preceding the publication, in 1886, of the paper on "Perforating Ulcer of the Vermiform Appendix" to the appearance in 1911 of the essay on "Zabdiel

Boylston, Inoculator, and the Epidemic of Small Pox in Boston in 1721,"—his last considerable contribution to medical literature,—this library was the frequent and often the prolonged witness of his patient labors, furnishing the cruder materials of medical observation and record to be transformed by his persistent study, close reasoning, successful ingenuity and terse English into the more perfected products of medical thought and science.[32]

Charles Pickering Putnam, another founder who had been a member of the governing body since 1877, died on April 22, 1914. For thirty-five years he was the mainspring behind the Directory of Nurses, which dominated this lucrative service in the area (and kept its sponsor's head above the financial tide) until the advancing professionalism of nursing produced competitors and finally, in 1911, the profession's own plan for a rival central directory. The business of the Library's agency declined markedly. The handwriting was on the wall. Immediately after Dr. Putnam's death the Directory was consigned to the house committee which, foreseeing a deficit, condemned it to euthanasia on December 31, 1914. Part of the Directory's ground floor quarters fronting on the Fenway was taken over by Dr. Farlow as the Librarian's first office since the founding; the inevitable steel stacks found their way into the rest of it, followed by 12,000 volumes of periodicals.[33]

The gaps in each day's post from overseas were unneeded reminders of the deepening war in Europe. In 1913 the BML offered 235 German journals in its current file; in 1916 it offered none. Short coal supplies after America's entry closed the Library on winter Mondays and evenings, and the tempers of the staff shortened with them. Could the clamor of the suffragettes have penetrated the brick of even 8 The Fenway? Dr. Richard G. Wadsworth had succeeded his late father on the governing committee and was delegated in March 1917 to the uncomfortable assignment of speaking to Assistant Librarian Ballard about complaints of female employees of his "alleged discourtesy," and drew from him a "promise to do better."[34]

That was not the end of it. Ought Mrs. E. F. Crosby in cataloguing get a raise? Dr. Wadsworth consulted C. K. Bolton, Librarian of the Athenaeum, reported back to the committee on library and finance, "and the question of employing college-bred women in place of the old retainer class as employees was discussed in its many bearings."[35] Twelve months elapsed, and the issue resolved itself. Mrs. Crosby and the indispensable Mrs. Collins threatened to quit unless they were raised, and raised they were, Mrs. Crosby to $960 a year, Mrs. Collins to $1125.

Dr. Farlow's retirement from practice in 1916 freed up all the time he wanted to give to the Library and to ponder the request of Dr. John Rührah of Baltimore in December 1917 that he complete a questionnaire on its history for inclusion in a treatise on the genus *bibliotheca medica* in America. He did more. He sat down and wrote *The History of the Boston Medical Library* and published it out of his own pocket, all before the Armistice.

With the end of the first great war of the twentieth century, *normalcy* (but never again normality) returned, and two voids were at least partly filled. Within a few months the Library had gathered in nearly complete sets of most of the foreign periodicals which had been interned, although Dr. Farlow mourned in his 1918 report that "I am afraid that many old friends have gone, to resume no more. Some of the journals remind one of a bear just finishing hibernation, so much have they lost of their pre-war thickness."

The other void, left by an insufficiency of funds, was the empty elevator well which the decrepit and dyspneic who had not gone off to camp or France had to haul themselves up around by stairs to attend meetings in Ware Hall. Their wheezings excited the sympathy of Mrs. Farlow. While her husband was producing his *History* at his expense, she had an elevator installed at hers. And that is how the Boston Medical Library got a much-needed lift at the end of the war.

7

Love's Labour's Lost

1919 · 1921

> I cannot quite see what is the matter with Medicine in general at this moment throughout the country. . . I have never seen anything that even approached the present state of excitement and unrest and unsteadiness in most places. I heard a very distinguished man say the other day that Harvard seemed to be the only medical school of importance in the country that was not having a brain storm.
> Dean David L. Edsall, May 26, 1921.[1]

The first annual meeting of the Boston Medical Library after the Armistice was four days before the opening of the peace conference in Paris, on January 14, 1919. George Brune Shattuck made it the occasion to mind the example of David Williams Cheever, upon the approach of *his* seventy-fifth birthday, and resigned the presidency. With that seemliness which had marked his editorship of the *Boston Medical and Surgical Journal*, Dr. Shattuck permitted his term of thirteen years to equal but not to exceed the tenure of Dr. Holmes, although he rather surpassed the old man in diligence, missing but six of the 143 meetings at which his office claimed his presence.

His successor was George Howard Monks, the vice president who had shouldered the grim burden of trying to raise money for to raise a stack building atop the stunted basement addition after his retirement in 1914 as Surgeon-in-Chief at Boston City Hospital and Lecturer at Harvard Medical School. After his graduation from the School in 1880 Monks trained for four years in Europe, which he topped off with a diploma from the Royal College of Surgeons. His best known contribution to surgery was the Mütter Lecture at the Philadelphia College of Physicians, "Studies on the Surgical Anatomy of the Small Intestine and Its Mesentery," in 1904. His service to Harvard and education lodged higher in the alimentary tract, thirty years of it for the Harvard Dental School, where he was still Professor of Oral Surgery. A connoisseur not alone of the animate, the sixth president of the Library was a sculptor not unrecognized, as deft in clay as flesh.

Less than six months after taking titular charge of the overstuffed and underfunded storehouse of medical knowledge on the Fenway, Dr. Monks was presented with an intriguing proposition. The new president of the Massachusetts Medical Society, Dr. Alfred Worcester, approached him in June of 1919 on behalf of two of the three owners of the *Boston Medical and Surgical Journal*, Doctors Joel E. Goldthwait and Hugh Williams (the third, Edward C. Streeter, was on the BML's governing committee); they wished to dispose of their shares to the Library and have it assume entire charge as publisher. The *Journal* had come perilously close to going under during the war, and the outlook was grim.

So offhandedly had the world's oldest medical periodical in continuous publication been bandied from owner to owner, editor to editor and press to press in arriving at the distinction, the wonder is that it did. Editor and contributor over the years had relied on the resources of the BML during the Library's first and second incarnations, and occasionally presided over them too. John Collins Warren and James Jackson and most of the other founders of the *New England Journal of Medicine and Surgery and the Collateral Branches of Science* in 1812 had been active in getting up the Library in 1905. The first secretary of the BML, John G. Coffin, was editor of *The Boston Medical Intelligencer* in 1828 when after five years of publication it was bought by Warren, John Ware and Walter Channing for $600 and merged with its only competitor under Warren's editorship as the *Boston Medical and Surgical Journal.*

For the next ninety years two dozen editors—most of them distinguished Boston clinicians—singly and jointly and with a range of taste and talent for the task got out some 4700 numbers in various formats with the help or hindrance of nine commercial publishers from about as many locations. From 1831 to 1873, D. Clapp and Company was proprietor as well. In that year John Collins Warren, William L. Richardson, George C. Shattuck, B. E. Cotting and Henry W. Williams purchased the *Journal* and returned it to professional ownership. In 1875 they chose H. O. Houghton publisher, then Houghton Mifflin in 1880, Cupples, Upham and Company in 1885 (proprietors of the Old Corner Bookstore), D. C. Heath in 1906 and W. M. Leonard in 1910.

Warren and Richardson had been joined in ownership by Frederick C. Shattuck, brother of George (who had retired in 1912 after thirty-one years as editor and was currently President of the BML), when they sold the *Journal* in 1914 to Goldthwait, Williams and Streeter. The first order of business before the new owners was a proposal just advanced by the Massachusetts Medical Society on the initiative of its president, Dr. Walter P. Bowers, a Clinton general practitioner, that the *Boston Medi-*

cal and Surgical Journal consent to be its official organ—or *mouthpiece*, as Secretary Burrage persisted in calling it. The proprietors were glad to oblige.

Dr. Robert M. Green agreed reluctantly in 1915 to be editor, less motivated, probably, by his Harvard *summa cum laude* in English than by the fact that his Grandfather John Ware was a co-founder. Green had little time for the job, and so many subscribers and contributors marched off to war that his *Journal* very nearly collapsed completely. With the end of the fighting in Europe, a new look at the *Journal* seems to have convinced its owners that it had reached the end of the line under private financing. Dr. Goldthwait tried and failed to bring off a merger of all the medical periodicals of New England. Then in some desperation he advanced his proposition that the Boston Medical Library throw open its doors and take in an old friend out of the cold.

The suggestion that the Boston Medical Library and the *Boston Medical and Surgical Journal*, whose beginnings and courses had such common root, should unite in fact for the advancement of medical knowledge, was a tempting one. President Monks agitated over it all that first summer of peace. Nevertheless, although neither his conclusions nor the reasoning behind the decision of the committee on library and finance appear in the minutes of October 20, 1919, the committee voted after a long and probably hot discussion that "it is *not* for the best interests of the Library to adopt the suggestion." Insufficient office space at 8 The Fenway and the chilling prospect of perennial subsidy out of funds then nonexistent may be presumed to have been high among the negative considerations which diverted the Library from the hazardous byway of medical journalism.

The *Journal*'s future looked bleak indeed, when suddenly it was assured.

In 1921, again between the push and pull of Dr. Bowers, the Medical Society purchased the *Journal* outright, and "Uncle Walter," as he was affectionately addressed by his younger associates, was cajoled against his inclination into the managing editorship. Office room was applied for, but the BML had less to spare than ever, and editorial supervision continued from the plant of the Jamaica Printing Company in Boston.[2]

Hardly had the Library reluctantly rejected the role of foster parent to the *Journal* when the strains of a familiar siren song were wafted Fensward on the westerly breeze, that it rejoin the warm, maternal, academic fold as stepchild of the Harvard Medical School. Actually, a union was proposed, but with strong oedipal undertones. It had been supposed that such fantasies collapsed when Professor Archie

Coolidge's trial blimp was shot down in 1914. Well, there had been a war which coincided with a watershed; all was ferment, discontent and contention; the School in 1918 had a new Dean, David Linn Edsall, as the Library had a new President; and not least, Dr. Farlow's innocent *History*, an unknowing Trojan horse, had brought fresh reinforcements to the Muddy River front where all had been quiet for four years.

Among the readers of the *History* was Dr. Frederic T. Lewis, Associate Professor of Embryology and chairman *pro tem* of the School's committee on library during the short war absence of its ensconced chief, Elliott Joslin. On September 18, 1919 Lewis directed a letter to President Emeritus Eliot inquiring if he had ever expressed an opinion about the relations of the Boston and Harvard medical libraries. "It seems clearly desirable that these two libraries should be brought together," he wrote, "as they were at the beginning, and that the medical books formerly belonging to the college or to its professors should not be housed a mile away from the place where they are so often needed. There are, however, many difficulties in this medical-library problem, and it would help if I knew more of the former attitude of the School than is presented in Dr. Farlow's book which, of course, is from the separatist standpoint."[3]

President Eliot replied from his summer home at Northeast Harbor, Maine, on September 21 that he hadn't ventured anything recently on the subject, but "is it probable or supposable that the Boston Medical Library Association should get a new library building on land close to the Medical School and the Hospitals which surround it? That I think would be the best solution of the problem you are considering."[4]

Thus armed by the highest authority, "Duffy" Lewis (every Lewis these days was so nicknamed after the famous Boston Red Sox outfielder) drafted an article which he rather undiplomatically entitled "The Future of the Boston Medical Library,"[5] wherein he advanced the bare-knuckled proposition that the Library should abandon all plans for expansion on the Fenway and move to new and larger quarters near the School and hospitals in that area it was no longer able to serve adequately. The first Boston Medical Library was a creature of Harvard, he argued, and when its reincarnation arose in 1875 "it was never imagined that the library might stand in the way of progress in the School. On the contrary it was the evident purpose of the founders to serve their University and its graduates by providing, not only for them but for the entire profession, an unrivaled library of their own, wholly independent of the School, but never losing sight of its interests." It was on this presumption, Lewis contended, that quantities of volumes were deposited by the School and College libraries, and his personal library by Dr.

Holmes, all to the detriment of the School, whose current efforts to consolidate a central library out of the departmental collections were in his view futile.

The embryologist let escape a hint of what was nettling him: the odyssey of a histology instructor on a semantic search after something or other which led him through four department libraries at the School and ended, finally, at the Boston Medical Library in a volume containing a Harvard bookplate.

"It would seem therefore," he advanced, "that the Medical Library might profitably appoint a committee to consider the problem further and devise a plan of removal and enlargement which would be to its own advantage, and at the same time be a project in which the Medical School and the adjacent hospitals might cooperate and bring to realization. Otherwise there may be an inglorious outcome of the devoted efforts which have produced the Medical Library, by ending in competition with the University from which it came."

The author conceded that his plan would remove the BML even farther from the Tufts Medical School, though not so separated as it was then from Harvard, while "for practitioners it would doubtless seem more distant, though not so far away as the Fenway site was regarded at the time of its selection."

Dr. Lewis submitted his article to Dean Edsall and Assistant Dean Worth Hale (who approved it "heartily") and to three members of the committee on library, S. Burt Wolbach and Percy G. Stiles, who okayed it without comment, and David Cheever, son of the late BML president, who passed it without his full endorsement. On December 4 he gave copies to Dr. Farlow and Dr. Green, the editor of the *Boston Medical and Surgical Journal*. President Monks read it and dismissed it as "propaganda."[6] Green accepted it for publication, but when Lewis, who was himself a Fellow, asked James Ballard for the mailing list of the members so he could circulate reprints to them, the Assistant Librarian refused him, and Farlow was able to talk the editor out of his decision to run the article.[7]

What the rejected author did not know was that the officers of the Library were at this moment reaffirming their commitment to their Fenway location, and that Morton Prince, who had initially taken charge of the attempt to build the stack addition in 1913 and was now retired from the Tufts faculty, had been sounding out a trustee he knew at the Carnegie Corporation about a construction grant for the BML; he had been advised to hold off and apply again later in the light of possible policy changes occasioned by the death of Andrew Carnegie on August 11, 1919.[8]

Lewis's protests to Farlow were in vain. On the fifteenth of December the Librarian brought the suppressed article before the committee on library and finance, which took no action. The annual meeting on January 13, 1920 adopted new by-laws, returning to the executive committee form of government, this time around to consist of the officers, chairmen of the committees on medical and social meetings and on membership and elections, and three at-large members, eliminating the library and finance committee and the council of the corporation. On the nineteenth, the newly formed executive committee agreed without dissent that the Lewis scheme "can lead to no practical result" and tabled it. Or so it supposed.

Although he was unwell and had been displaced as chairman of the committee on library by the return of Dr. Joslin, Dr. Lewis pressed on. In April he moved to enlist President A. Lawrence Lowell of Harvard, in a letter revealing more than a little prophetic insight.

April 10, 1920.

My dear President Lowell:

I had hoped for an opportunity to talk with you about the Medical Library situation, but as it has not appeared, I am venturing to write of what I regard as a most urgent matter. There are, of course, various views as to the value of medical libraries to medical schools, and the successors in the faculty of those who allowed our books to go do not consider this library question vital at all. Some believe in private libraries; others in private libraries supported by school funds; still others in slightly larger libraries to serve a few departments with their students. Of late a central library has had its advocates, well pleased with throwing together very skillfully several ill-adapted rooms, and in starting out to accomplish what the Medical Library has already done. The possibility of having the Medical Library move so that the school may have close by for its use a better collection of books than is available to any other medical school in the country appeals to me as worthy of great effort. It seems to appeal also to Drs. Edsall, Bradford, Tyzzer, Joslin, and some others with whom I have discussed it, and especially to Dr. J. C. Warren.

President Farlow of the Medical Library said that it would be good to have the school and the library near together and suggested that the school should move to the library. He said that you had found that not all desirable mergers could be brought about; and evidently resented Dr. Cushing's proposition which he implied was an invitation to annihilate the medical library.[9] In spite of the opposition of the officers of the library I do not regard the situation as hopeless, and offer the following suggestions.

1. That the medical school purchase a large lot on the corner of Pasteur and Longwood Avenues, for the purpose of building a library. This lot will certainly be needed for school purposes, even if no library should be built, and since the income from the houses upon it will pay the taxes, as I am told, it would seem not unwise to acquire it as soon as possible. A fine lot set apart for a library will

cause the medical library to give serious attention to the situation, such as it has not yet done.

2. That the medical school seek the gift of a fine library building, which in time it ought to obtain. If the Medical Library could be invited to an equally good building but larger than the one it now has, there would be a reasonable possibility of inducing it to move.

A very important consideration would be the sale of their present building. Dr. Farlow was pleased to say that the Historical Society which might have bought the building has decided to enlarge in other ways, but Dr. Warren is chairman of the Committee of the Historical Society having charge of this matter and he has told me that the Historical Society is still a possible purchaser.

Whenever I have talked with Dr. Farlow, he has asked, "What has the medical school to offer?" It seems that it is now time to act, so that there may be something to offer which will compel the medical library to think seriously of its future.

I trust that the Overseers and all others interested in the Harvard Medical School may consider the Library situation, and that something may be planned commensurate with the dignity of the school; the present makeshifts certainly are not.

Regretting that illness prevents me from discussing this farther, and from meeting the Overseers on their next visit, I am,

Respectfully yours,
Frederic T. Lewis[10]

A week later and President Lowell replied:

April 17, 1920.

Dear Dr. Lewis:

Many thanks for your letter about the Medical Library. That the Medical School ought to have a Library of its own, or one in close proximity, is wholly evident; and the best solution would, no doubt, be for the Medical Society Library to establish itself close to the Medical School. I am afraid this will be very difficult to bring about; but if it cannot I see no alternative but to have the Medical School create a library of its own. I wish I knew how we could bring some influence to bear upon the Medical Society Library. I am advised that probably Dr. J. Collins Warren has more influence with them than anybody else.

Yours very truly,
A. Lawrence Lowell[11]

In going over the Dean to the President with his campaign, Professor Lewis seems not to have realized that it was already yielding first fruits. Three days previously, on April 7, Dr. Edsall wrote Dr. Henry S. Pritchett, president of the Carnegie Foundation for the Advancement of Teaching and the man behind Abraham Flexner's explosive exposé of medical education, sounding him out if the fund might support a merger of the libraries at the School. "I have no authority at all to speak for the Boston Medical Library," the Dean admitted, "and do not therefore know what action they may take concerning the matter. . . The Boston Medical Library already has, I believe, some building fund but not sufficient. Just what it is I cannot state. I should not like to take the matter up with them unless there was some reasonable prospect of its meeting favorable consideration from the Carnegie Corporation. . ."[12] Dr. Pritchett replied on April 16 that while the amalgamation of the two was "a result well worth bringing about if it can be done," the Corporation was low on funds for the balance of the year, and besides, was getting a new president, Dr. James R. Angell, on whom the decision would fall after he had acquainted himself with the job; he advised Edsall to bide his time.[13]

This overture suited the committee on library, which on May 17 asked Chairman Joslin "to express to the Dean the Committee's appreciation and approval of his efforts to bring about the union of the Boston Medical Library and the Library of the Harvard Medical School upon a basis which would be mutually advantageous to the patrons of each institution. . . The Committee feels that one large library which would accomodate all could be created and would serve as a distinctive feature before the country of Boston's eminence in medicine."[14]

Ten days later the Dean got more encouragement than he had expected in a letter from Dr. Henry A. Christian at the National Research Council, an old friend and a predecessor in the deanship, who had spoken with Dr. Angell and sized him up as "not unfavorable to such a proposition. . . I assume that you would first have to get the assent of the Medical Library to move and to consolidation with the Medical School, then estimate the resources in sight for a new plant, the size of the plant that is needed, and the additional money that will be required, before you will be in a position to submit the thing to the Carnegie Corporation. I should judge that there was enough possibility of favorable consideration to justify doing this amount of work. . . I would rather think that the idea of economy and improvement by consolidation and the value of such a plant to the improvement of both medical education and investigation on the one hand, and medical practice on the other in furnishing better facilities to the local physicians, is what would have the strongest appeal."[15]

However, Edsall had so much more pressing on his mind than a new library that for the remainder of 1920 he made no further moves. The absence of any action provoked Professor Lewis to carry his crusade to the medical faculty at a meeting on December 3, when he reviewed his case and renewed his plea that the University buy the land at Longwood and Louis Pasteur avenues. In response to President Lowell's inquiry as to what he proposed should be done, he "expressed a desire," according to the minutes, "that the need of a considerable gift for a library should be recognized as an important and immediate need of the School, by those in a position to influence the purpose of gifts; since at any time a bequest to the Medical Library for enlarging its present quarters may produce a very difficult situation.'[16]

Apparently this reactivated the Dean. On January 5, 1921 he wrote Angell suggesting that they meet the following week in New York to determine if the possibility of Carnegie assistance was real enough for him then to take it up with the BML people. Edsall wrote that he hadn't talked with them directly, but "some persons close to their councils have informed me that they thought they would be glad to consider it in a thoroughly friendly spirit if it would be a means of helping them financially to accomplish the developments that they need."[17]

But even as the unsuspecting Harvard Dean was resuming his circumspections, Dr. Prince of Tufts was working to advance unilaterally the cause of the Medical Library. In mid-January Prince persuaded Pritchett to present its building needs to the trustees of the parent Carnegie Corporation. His move drew from the surprised Dr. Angell the almost immediate counterquery: had Prince consulted with Edsall about the medical library situation in Boston?[18]

The question put the Library leaders on their guard. Dr. Harold C. Ernst, the retiring Professor of Bacteriology at Harvard, had already hinted broadly to his friend Farlow that something was in the wind at the School. Ernst was opposed to the Lewis scheme, favored the existing combination of departmental libraries for the faculty and a small central one for the students. . . nevertheless, would the BML consider moving near the School, autonomously, if upwards of $400,000 fell into its treasury? No, said Farlow—we'd use it to expand where we are. On February 2 Ernst told the Librarian "the possible gift of 3 or $400,000 was on condition of a merger of the Med. Sch. Libr. & B.M.L. with moving the latter to near the Med. Sch. & in case there was no merger the gift would lapse. He did not say that any money had been promised, but I inferred that perhaps application had been made to the Carnegie Corpor. by Dr. Edsall as Dean. Dr. Ernst does not believe in this at all & considers it mistaken and expensive policy. He suggested using the Rotch Infants Hosp. (now bankrupt) as a sort of central libr. for the school, the present stacks to be retained in their present situation. Dr. E. thinks many at the school are in favor of a large library. Prest Lowell probably does not wish it."[19]

Farlow sought reassurance the next day from Joslin, who "told me that he knew nothing about using the Infants Hosp. for a library.[20] He said there was room for 100,000 vols. in the basement of the present libr.

bldg. & was enough for many years. The ideal thing, according to him, would be a consolidation of libraries, but this would cost 1 or $2,000,000 and unless this money could be found, which he thought doubtful, he considered that the only thing to do was to stay as we were."[21]

Another who found himself uncomfortably in the middle was Dr. J. Collins Warren. He had given Lewis the impression of his support; now he was braced at the Massachusetts Historical Society by the Librarian from next door, who reported in his *Medical Library Notes* on February 12:

He said he hoped I didn't think he was conspiring against me but he feared I might have heard that he was interested in Dr. Lewis's scheme for a merger of libraries. Dr. L. had read a paper at the Med. Sch. which had caused some interest. He, Dr. W., said he saw no way of such a merger & did not know where a million dollars could come from. He asked what Dr. Chadwick had thought of a consolidation with the Med. Sch. libr. & I said he was much opposed. The B.M.L. should not be attached to any one school, but should be of use to all. Dr. W. thinks that is a correct view of the case.

I should think the Carnegie Corp. had been approached (several years ago) with the hope of getting $500,000 for a big libr. for the H.M.S. & the B.M.L. combined, but nothing came of it.

The fact is that even then the game was up. The Dean's antennae had picked up the danger signals, and on February 9 he had blown the whistle in a letter to Dr. Angell:

I am writing simply to say that I do not think it is wise at present to attempt to carry any further the Library developments that I discussed with you. It could not be done without an effort to raise a considerable amount of money, of which obviously from my conversation with you a considerable share would have to come from here, and two other matters of such pressing importance have come since that time that I think all our efforts should be devoted to them for a little time to come. I am also of the opinion that the views of the officers of the Boston Medical Library expressed to me concerning the probability of their undertaking a development and a move represent to such an uncertain degree the opinion of their body in general that it is questionable on that account whether anything should be done about it at present. I shall therefore at present not press the matter any further.[22]

The Carnegie president agreed to strike the Harvard library from his list and volunteered the tip that "you are perhaps aware that, after your interview with me, Dr. Morton Prince presented considerations relating to the Boston Medical Library which I felt should be handled in connection with your proposal, if possible."[23]

The suspicion at 8 The Fenway that Dean Edsall was a competitive supplicant was strengthened by President Angell's warning to Dr. Prince at the end of February, namely, that if there are rival medical libraries in Boston, the foundation will come to the assistance of neither. Unaware that he already had done so, Dr. Monks wondered how the Dean might be induced to withdraw his horns. Dr. Farlow told him "I thought Dr. E. would find it difficult and unwise to say that the H.M.S. Libr. would give up its wish to become a large library, and agree to limit itself to the limited needs of a med. school." Perhaps Dr. Warren, with his appreciation of the aims of the BML, could influence the Dean or President Lowell. But when Farlow took this tack a couple of days later, Warren advised lying low for a while on the hunch that nothing would come of the School's library plans anyway.[24]

Finally, at the insistence of Dr. Angell, Dr. Monks arranged a summit meeting with Dean Edsall on March 17. Monks reported the gist of it to Farlow, who recorded:

> Dr. E. said there should be no rivalry, that the Sch. Libr. was small & was for different purpose. Some time they would need a larger building. He will write to Dr. Angell that there is no rivalry & will send a copy of this letter to Dr. Monks. He says Dr. Lewis is not well and does not have any following in his ideas about a fusion & moving to near the Med. School.[25]

In view of his own machinations toward precisely that end, Edsall's disavowal of intent and dismissal of Lewis as a serious factor in the pursuit of fusion (if he was quoted correctly in this second-hand account) was less than ingenuous, most particularly in the light of Dr. Joslin's choice of this moment to define the issue, and then to skirt it adroitly:

> March 22, 1921.
>
> David L. Edsall, Dean
> Harvard Medical School
>
> My dear Dean:
>
> Your effort to bring about the amalgamation of the libraries of the Boston Medical Library and of the Harvard Medical School in a situation accessible to the school by the solicitation of funds from the Carnegie Foundation [26] is appreciated by the Committee on Library. It is evident that you made a forcible presentation of the matter, because now the Carnegie Foundation asks why this is not to be brought about, when an appropriation is requested for the expansion of one of those Institutions alone.
>
> It is manifest that if the Carnegie Foundation should become interested in Libraries in Boston, it would approve of a project drawn upon broad lines. Should it decide to make a grant for this purpose it would probably prefer to give $500,000 for a combined library rather than $100,000 for a single enterprise. The subject, therefore, becomes one of fundamental importance, and with such a possibility in mind the President and Corporation might conclude to make an offer to duplicate such a gift from the Carnegie Foundation so that its Medical School would have the prestige of facilities for books superior to that of any Medical School in the Country and perhaps in the world.
>
> If such an arrangement should be culminated, in the end the Boston Medical Library would receive ten to one, or even more in endowment than by continuing in its present isolated position.

Perhaps the most serious objection of all to the expansion of the Boston Medical Library on its own account at the present time is that thereby there will be created two rival libraries in Boston. Already the library of the Medical School is as large as that of the Boston Medical Library half a generation ago, and its development has been proportionately more rapid. In other words, unless there is to be a fusion of the two libraries near enough to the Medical School for the use of Harvard students there will inevitably be much duplication, and not a little waste. Even though the two institutions may work most happily together [the prevention of] the growth of a rival library cannot be avoided, because the Harvard Medical School cannot refuse the acceptance of gifts of books for the benefit of its students.

Your attention is also called to the peculiar situation which now exists between the Library of Harvard University and the Boston Medical Library. Some 5,000 books belonging to the University, many of which bear the book plates of Harvard University, are now deposited in the Boston Medical Library. The University claims the right to withdraw these books, a considerable number of which are needed for work in its departments; the Boston Medical Library on the other hand claims these books as an outright gift, is perfectly willing to loan but unwilling to return them. If the Medical School now favors the abandonment of the plan for a common library and seeks to perpetuate the growth of the Boston Medical Library it would hardly be consistent for it to request the return of these books. This question should be settled by legal representatives of the two Institutions examining the facts in order to determine what is right. It is a serious matter for Harvard University to lose property entrusted to its care. Lawyers and not doctors or professors should arrange a settlement so that the harmonious relations existing between the two claimants may be preserved.

In consideration of the outline above submitted I would ask as Chairman of the Committee on Library that before any step is taken which involves the future policy of the Harvard Medical School and of the University as well, the Administrative Board give an opportunity for those interested to present the case and for the Librarian of the University, the President and Corporation to express their opinion.

While the Committee on Library believes the interests of this community would be best served by one large library of national importance, situated near the Medical School, in which collections of the Boston Medical Library and the Harvard Medical School could be concentrated, if the large expenditure involved is an absolute bar to the attainment of this purpose in the opinion of the Corporation, the Committee would be glad to see the School and University join with the Boston Medical Library in soliciting from the public the perpetuation and growth of the Boston Medical Library on its present site.

Respectfully yours,
Elliott P. Joslin[27]

Professor Lewis did not share in the magnanimous recommendation of the committee on library, if indeed he participated in it. He wrote President Lowell, his last resort, a furious letter:

Philadelphia
March 24, 1921

My dear President Lowell,

Just before I left Boston to attend the session of anatomists, Dr. Joslin informed me by telephone of the important meeting which I suppose has taken place between the Dean and Dr. Prince, in regard to supporting the appeal of the Boston Medical Library for Carnegie Funds. I was told that our Administrative Board was not opposed to this appeal, and that the Dean had decided not to "push" his plans for bringing the Library near the School. In this situation, which seems a final move on the part of a shrewd and united organization to outwit and outplay the University, I hope that you and the Corporation may exert a deciding influence.

I cannot reconcile myself to the state of affairs in which the heirlooms and treasures of the Medical School are held by an alien institution a mile away. With these are costly files which now cannot be duplicated and which the School would have secured had it not regarded the Medical Library—as in fact it was—an affiiliated body with common interests and purpose. Such files are needed for research.

I cannot agree with Professor Ernst that the question is simply one of money—else the Medical Library would not have reported to the Carnegie Trustees that the Library was unanimously against removal. It is not improbable that certain disappointed Harvard men who have been in control of the Library are not as ingenuous as Dr. Ernst would have it appear. Why should the Harvard Medical School endorse the plans of those who have given the wishes of the School not an iota of favorable consideration?

Believing that you are in a position to prevent this and that providing an adequate library is a vital issue for the School I am

Sincerely yours,
Frederic T. Lewis[28]

Within the week Professor Lewis had the answer he was hoping for:

March 28, 1921

Dear Dr Lewis:

Your letter of March 24th has come. It seems to me very unfortunate that the Boston Medical Library and the Medical School should not get together. Otherwise it seems to me inevitable that we shall have two rival libraries, to a great extent duplicates, within a quarter of a mile of each other. It does not seem to me that we ought to promote what would seem to be inevitably an unfortunate situation.

Very truly yours,
A. Lawrence Lowell[29]

To his Dean the President of Harvard communicated in like vein the same day:

March 28, 1921

Dear Dr Edsall:

I have been thinking over your letter about the Medical Library and consulting with Professor A. C. Coolidge. It does not seem to either of us that the suggestion of helping to build up the Boston Medical Library where it is, and of having some method of delivering books at the Medical School, would be satisfactory. It would inevitably result in the building up of two rival libraries a quarter of a mile apart, which would, to a great extent, duplicate one another. It does not seem to me, therefore, that we ought to help to bring about that condition. I return Dr Joslin's letter.

Very truly yours,
A. Lawrence Lowell[30]

President Lowell, who has been described as a *pragmatic relativist*,[31] soon found occasion to assist the dog up into the manger, as related to Librarian Farlow two weeks hence by Secretary Burrage, who "told me Dr. Monks had been to see him and said that Dr. Edsall had not sent to Dr. Monks a copy of the letter he was to send to Dr. Angell of the Carnegie Corporat. but the question of writing such a letter had been brought up at the Harv. Med. Sch. Faculty meeting & referred to Mr. Lowell & Prof. Coolidge & Prest. Lowell was opposed to sending any letter saying that the Med. Sch. renounced its right or was willing to withdraw, because it might be desirable later to have rights."[32]

For the rest of 1921 the Boston Medical Library remained in a state of unhopeful suspense, buoyed briefly by Angell's encouragement of Morton Prince late in April to apply again at the end of the year. Then in May descended a double blow: Prince's fall-back overtures to the Rockefeller Foundation were rejected, and Dr. Angell was called to the presidency of Yale. Instead of gifts at Yuletide, Henry S. Pritchett sent a Scroogian greeting. . . the Library was out in the cold. . . the departed Angell had spent or committed Carnegie funds far into the future, and the goose would be barren of golden eggs for a long time to come.[33]

When Harvard acquired the land at the north corner of Longwood and Louis Pasteur avenues—but for the student dormitory which Harold S. Vanderbilt largely financed, and not a library—Frederic Lewis was bitterly disappointed and remonstrated with Dr. Joslin, who was taking the lead in it as president of the Harvard Medical Alumni Association. Lewis was still a member of the committee on library and scolded his chairman that "in the future our failure to use to the utmost the opportunity to secure and develop. . . a library will be regarded as showing an incomprehensible lack of judgment and foresight. With the example of the Widener Library before us, which is to the College no more and no less than what a medical library should be to this school, I cannot understand the enthusiasm for dormitories to the exclusion of all consideration of this subject. I fancy that the founders of Harvard College, at least, would have provided a library first and comforts and conveniences later."[34]

With a trace of testiness, Dr. Joslin responded that the Alumni and the Aesculapian Club would back a dormitory but not a library, while among the faculty "there was no enthusiasm for a library in the remote future compared with a dormitory in the immediate present."[35]

Without much doubt, anything less expedient than a modest shift in emphasis away from departmental libraries and towards a student reading room or two was low among Dean Edsall's postwar priorities for the Harvard Medical School. When he met the hostility of the Boston Medical Library to another westward move and even the semblance of affiliation, and a dearth of ready funds to finance it, he quietly backed off, for his plant was run down, applicants as never before were clamoring for admission, he was under pressure to increase the enrollment, curricular and methodological reforms were on his mind, a dormitory was being agitated, the School of Public Health was in conception, and every other school and teaching hospital in the country seemed bent on raiding his faculty.

Understandably, the insufficiencies of their piecemeal library were felt most keenly, if subjectively, by the preclinical faculty at Harvard. The 1919-1921 attempt to try to get 8 The Fenway to roll obediently up Avenue Louis Pasteur was notable neither for finesse nor for a spirit of altruism toward the larger medical community. Possibly the outcome would have been otherwise if the Harvard medical establishment, for all its possessiveness, had something to offer, as Dr. Farlow had so blandly challenged it. Most remarkable through it all, perhaps, was the combative clairvoyance of that honorless prophet, Frederic Thomas Lewis.

For the third time in thirty-eight years, the python had choked on the porker, and the more or less friendly rivals relaxed again into guarded symbiosis.

8

Too Much Too Soon, Too Little Too Late

1919 · 1930

A landmark, or rather another high water mark, was attained in 1919 with a surge of postwar acquisitions which lifted the book level at the Boston Medical Library above a hundred thousand, to 102,433 by catalogue count, pamphlets to 62,982. All this included neither the duplicate library of 10,000 volumes, nor the 60,000-odd theses hoarded in the cellar awaiting cataloguing, nor some 8,000 volumes received from the Essex Institute of Salem—a dusty cache of early and mid-nineteenth century books, pamphlets, journals, autographs and miscellany deposited there long ago, mainly by the Essex South District Medical Society. In 1920 the Library joined the interlibrary loan network as a service to physicians outside the normal circulation area.

"James hinted that it might be a good idea to send someone to Europe to purchase med. books for the libr., meaning himself," Dr. Farlow jotted knowingly in his *Medical Library Notes* on February 12, 1919. And indeed, in the summer of 1920 Assistant Librarian Ballard crossed the Atlantic, at the expense of the Rockefeller Foundation for the ostensible purpose of enriching the Peking Medical School Library. However, in another pocket he held a credit of $10,000 from his employers in Boston. He returned that fall with $3000 unspent and nearly all the significant French and German medical works published during the Great War, having also managed on the side to carry out a purchasing assignment for the library of the Harvard Medical School. During the next two years several substantial private collections were gathered in from Germany, including Felix Droysen's on gynecology and obstetrics and Rudolph Kobert's on pharmacology and toxicology; so many bureaucratic obstacles were put in the way of the latter that the intervention of the State Department was required finally to pry it loose from the *dienstweg* of the Republic. Foreign exchange fluctuations heightened the gamble.

The economic climate of the early Twenties was no more favorable to moneyraising for completion of the basement addition than 1914, and for lack of anything more concrete to create, Edward C. Streeter and Malcolm Storer of the executive committee were designated in March of 1921 to select a third with the object of stimulating interest in the Library's esoterica by organizing a society devoted to the history of medicine. They picked Harvey Cushing. It was agreed that J. Collins Warren was the man to be the first president, but he demurred, and when the Boston Medical History Club pulled itself together on October 20 at the home of its institutional parent, Dr. Cushing was in the chair, and Dr. Streeter was elected secretary-treasurer. Thereafter for a score or more of years the club met monthly for papers and talk during the season; by 1922 the subject in general and the magnetism of the president in particular had attracted a membership of 120.

Harvey Cushing's keenness for the past of the profession was as sharp as his bibliophilia and his every other cutting edge. He had been a Fellow of the Library since 1912, when he came back to Boston from Johns Hopkins to help create the new Peter Bent Brigham Hospital and to serve as its surgeon-in-chief and professor at Harvard, where he would literally if not nominally dominate the department and harass Dean Edsall with his demands that the Brigham be recognized as *the* teaching facility. During the war he organized Base Hospital Number 5 and took it to France, where he operated incessantly and to his physical cost in 1917 on shattered central nervous sytems. His reappearance at the Library was remarked with deference by the Librarian in June 1919: "Told Dr. Harvey Cushing that he might take out more than the usual number of books at a time while writing a monograph."[1]

Sir William Osler, who had profoundly influenced Cushing in the Baltimore days, died on December 29, 1919. At its annual meeting two weeks later the Library adopted a resolution drawn up by Dr. Streeter:

> *Whereas*, in the death of Sir William Osler this Library has suffered the loss of a great friend, who throughout his career did most generously support and further its development, giving timely encouragement to its Founders, inspiring its promoters in the succeeding forty-three years by every means in his power, by treasured advice to its committees, by many treasured gifts for its shelves, by not infrequent visits, more notably at the dedication of our present building and on the well-remembered occasion of his address on Thomas Linacre;
>
> And *Whereas*, William Osler was the first, and last surviving Honorary Member on the roll of our Library, in conferring of which distinction in 1911 this Corporation will never cease to take pride;
>
> Be it therefore *Resolved*, that the Officers and Members of the Boston Medical Library record their profound grief and sorrow over the loss of this beloved physician, their friend, one of the rarest, loveliest and best spirits that rolling time ever pressed from his vintage; exemplar of all that is highest in our humanity, whose sovereign mind, resilient to the last, fertilized Letters and the Sciences through half a century.[2]

Soon after her husband's death, Lady Osler asked Cushing to write his biography. He agreed and began his research almost immediately. On March 15, 1920 Farlow mentioned in his *Notes* that "Dr. Harvey Cushing tells me he has been asked to write a life of Dr. Osler & would like to see what letters we have of his. I got out some from the vault." For the most part of five years the neurosurgeon squeezed the great project into an already overflowing career. When *The Life of Sir William Osler*, in two volumes, appeared in 1925 it rewarded him with the Pulitzer Prize in biography.

While he was immersed in the Osler work "The Chief," who had a short fuse and was not used to a snuffing by anyone, came off second best in an encounter at the Library with one of the Boston Codmans, John S., a leading spirit in the New England Anti-Vivisectionist Society. It involved John Farlow and provided that mildest of men with some dry amusement. With a due sense of the historic import of the confrontation, he committed it to his *Notes*:

Dec. 10, 1921: John S. Codman has recently been at library looking up references to use in his anti-vivisection addresses. Today he came to the library, signed the book, made out slips for journals, & was reading at the table. Dr. Harvey Cushing came in to Holmes Hall to look up some references. He & the anti-vivis had been having some discussions in the papers about the anti-vivis opposition to the Red Cross during the war.[3]

When Dr. Cushing saw Mr. Codman reading at the table in Holmes Hall, he went up to Mr. Codman & asked him what he was doing there, whether he had permission to use the library. He said the library was not a public library, but was for the use of the medical profession that supported it, etc. He thought it very bad taste for any one to come to the library to get material to use against the medical profession. Mr. Codman said he had not special permission, but had understood the library was open to the public for the use of books & journals at the library, not, of course, to be taken out. He then went away.

I came to the libr. soon after this and saw Dr. Cushing looking over a number of books on the centre table. He told me that he wanted me to back him up, as he had insulted some one, referring to Mr. Codman & his remarks to Mr. C. He asked me if the library was public, as Mr. C. had claimed, or whether it was not private in the sense that non-members had to get permission to use it. He thought Harv. Med. students had to have a request or permit in order to use the books.

I said that the library was open to the public and no permission to consult books was needed; students (medical) were free to use it. I showed him the last paragraph in the Preface of the History of the B.M.L., where it was distinctly stated that the library was open to the public, and anyone might use it, whether a member of the libr., or the medical profession or not. He thought the funds to carry on the libr. were contributed by med. profession, which is true only to a small extent. He was evidently convinced that he had been mistaken about the library, and immediately wrote a note to Mr. Codman, saying he must apologize for his misunderstanding of the library rules, etc. . . This all occurred about 11 A.M.

At 1:45 P.M. he [Codman] called me up from W. Roxbury. . . He said he was to take part in a discussion at the Public Library on vivisection. He felt that some of the statements made by anti-vivis might be loose or not quite correctly quoted from medical writings, and he was desirous of checking up these matters by consulting the best books, which he supposed were in the B.M.L. Dr. Cushing questioned his right to use the library, and he went away. He now called me to find out what the situation was.

I told him that the libr. was open to the public, whether members of the med. profession or not. I knew that he had been to the library before, that he had signed the book and had conformed to the ordinary library rules about asking for books to use at the library. I said he had the same right to use the library as anyone else, and I should be glad to have him come there. Any help that he needed would gladly be given to him. We wished the libr. to be used as much as possible. I told him of the statement in the Preface to the Hist. of the Libr. He thanked me for my "courtesy."

The chiefs, and a few of the Indians too, found that they had to knuckle under to the even-handed custodianship of the Librarian. Farlow was approaching the end of his tenure in 1927 when a Beacon Street physician wrote him "protesting against allowing lawyers freedom of the library. He had been sued for malpractice and had seen the 'unscrupulous' lawyer for the plaintiff consulting books at the library. I replied that the libr. was open to all who complied with the rules & we had no way of finding out who are unscrupulous lawyers or what use our readers are to make of the information gained at the library."[4]

It was Farlow's unshakable conception of the Library's commitment to the medical profession and the public at large which the Harvard matchmakers had run up against:

We have calls from members of the bench and bar for references as to effects of poisons and injuries and the nature of different diseases, especially insanity, and our books are often produced in court. Of a less serious nature was a letter referred to me from a young woman who wished to know the difference between the breath of life and the heart beat. An actor asked for suggestions as to how to make himself up to represent a student much injured in the face in a duel. A book of plates showing some cases of facial mutilation resulting from the Great War was given to him, and this proved enough and more than enough for his purpose. . . I have seen in our halls men hostile to medicine and the medical profession using our books and trying to use arguments to use at the State House to defeat sane medical legislation. We lose nothing by our hospitality; by keeping on friendly terms with all we extend our reputation for public spirit and willingness to do our utmost for the advancement of medical science and the general welfare.[5]

If James Read Chadwick was the cavalier, the knight errant, of the Boston Medical Library, as Clarence Blake had described him—the creator who moulded it to the shape of the void his genius perceived—then John Woodford Farlow, his heir, was the consolidator, careful, courtly in his vandyke, quietly tailored, deliberate, precise, jealous of his inheritance and of its autonomy, its identity, its holdings. . . the

Lowell, so to speak, to the Eliot. Chadwick got up a library in the guise of a private club of his peers (otherwise it could not have succeeded, with or without academic connections) and invested it with his own fervor and with the spirit of his idol, Oliver Wendell Holmes. Farlow was its steward, caterer to the vagaries of the Fellows, guardian of the inner mysteries, polisher of the golden oak, arbiter of the domestic staff, custodian of the morals, pincher of the pennies, thread of its continuity from the Victorian heyday of his first association with it when Boston medicine was in the unwashed hands of those giants of Galenic authority, with their ample hypertensive waistcoats, their olympian visages, their septic beards, their flowing, brown-stained mustaches, through the revolution wrought by science and Flexner, a world war, a sundered society and a new and less certain art practised from a jangling flivver, to the jingle of the jazz age.

No very important doings at the Library escaped pinioning in the succession of cheap ruled notebooks, his *Medical Library Notes*, which John Farlow kept with the prim gossipry of an assiduous schoolgirl until his retirement in 1928. Every job aspirant came under his scrutiny—and, for a time, under the eye of Mrs. Farlow, generous donor of the elevator. Thus one January he brought home letters from applicants for a clerical position, and "Annie read the handwriting & I wrote down on envelopes." Eighteen months later. . . "James [always *James* Ballard the lay employee, never *Jim*, as in Jim Chadwick] sent me some of the letters from applicants which Annie read, to see what the handwriting showed."[6]

It is related that one young hopeful endowed with a possibly distracting figure was commanded to stroll through the hall for the Librarian's inspection, and if demure enough, his approval. Another, newly hired, turned up for work in a petticoat which rustled so distinctly and deliciously to her every movement that she was ordered home to change into something less swishy.

Once accepted, however, the staff found the Librarian a chief (Ballard was their foreman) of infinite concern and almost inexhaustible patience. How he fretted over every sniffle and fidget, and how they fretted him with their close-quartered abrasions! "Saw Miss Wyman, new secy for James. She has a table near radiator. I hope it is not too warm." One April he was left a note "complaining of Miss ____'s insolence & disagreeable attitude toward those in the catalog room." He spent a large part of three days trying to adjudicate the dispute. A week later, "had talk w. Mrs. ____ & Miss ____ about their trouble w. Miss ____ & I tried to get them to forget their past differences & be decent to each other. Then

Miss ____ & Miss ____ came to my room & I tried to make them establish more friendly relations. They all seem much upset & not inclined to forgive or forget." No doubt at seventy-three Dr. Farlow supposed he was entitled to respite from domestic strife. On another occasion, "had most insulting replies & talk, quite unprovoked, from ____, who seems to be lacking in control & perhaps unbalanced in his mind."[7]

The Librarian was deeply disturbed by the failing health in 1919 of Mrs. Elizabeth Collins, the faithful cataloguer who had given forty of her sixty-nine years to her job. Dr. Henry Jackson visited her at home and discussed her case with Dr. Farlow. . . "he thinks she should stay a long time in bed. He quoted Dr. F. Minot 'Never tell an old woman she will die or she will dance on your grave.' " The Librarian sent a personal check to pay for her nursing.[8] Mrs. Collins ailed for three years, loyally dragging herself in when she could but shouldn't, and died on September 1, 1922. Farlow wrote a warm tribute in the *Boston Medical and Surgical Journal*, accompanied by a resolution of the governing board that "her untiring devotion to the cause of medical literature, with its difficult questions of classification and cataloguing, has been of the greatest value to the medical profession; and the Executive Committee wishes to record its appreciation of the important part that she took in the growth of the library from its small beginnings in 1880 to its present influence in the community."[9]

To the fastidious Librarian the cellar of 8 The Fenway was subterra incognita, and he was content that it should remain so, with its floors settling under that glacier of frozen knowledge, passage twisting and hazardous through the canyons of uncatalogued books and pamphlets which stratified even the coal bins since the Library had converted to oil heat in 1923 "with the prospect of a sufficiency of fuel in the future and marked economy in running expense." Out of sight down here, out of mind. It was the janitor's domain. "Johnson's French bull dog (bitch) 'accouched' in basement near furnace" one January day. Another time, with admiration, he chronicled the doings below: "Many cockroaches in basement, wh. eat paste, etc. from books. Johnson got 2 cans of Columbian powder ($1 each) at Pierce's, wh. he scattered about. This killed the roaches. A man had offered to do the work for $100 & said it would take a month."[10]

Upstairs the company was more to Dr. Farlow's taste, as at the annual meeting in 1920, when refreshments included "some bottles of Pabst beer, wh. had been saved over" (meaning *over* the intervening Volstead Act). Good fellowship and good friends. . . "Dr. Joslin sent a barrel of very good russet apples to the libr. I sampled them."[11] Doubtless from the Joslin farm in Oxford. Bibliographically, the Fellows were not so obliging:

> A year ago I took the liberty of suggesting that members of the Library should make out lists of papers written by them, whether published or in manuscript, and should send a copy of such lists, with the date and place of publication of such papers to the Library for safe keeping and future reference. I am sorry to say that what I thought a very reasonable request fell on barren soil, as only one list was sent me out of 833 members. I am not discouraged and will repeat my request, knowing as I do the probable great value of such bibliographical information in the future.[12]

Twenty-five years the senior of his assistant librarian, Farlow maintained an avuncular watch over *James*. In 1922 Ballard finished thirty years with the BML, but he was only forty-four, having started as Dr. Brigham's errand and stack boy in 1892 at fourteen, lacking all but a month of the eighth grade. The Librarian inherited the precocious youngster from Chadwick in 1905, although by the Twenties it was questionable who had inherited whom. Ballard by then had risen by dint of an astounding course of applied self-education to a position of respect in the field of medical bibliography and was regarded by the physicians who employed him with a kind of esteem which now and again broke through the instinct to patronize a most useful man who some may have wished was a prodigy of their own making. This unschooled fellow who cultivated the history of medicine that he might know what to acquire for the Library (and what to discard) and who taught himself Latin, French, German, Hebrew, and late in life, Russian, and mastered the rare books marketplace, to know the nature and worth of what he was acquiring, grew so in stature that by middle age he was as well known around the world as he was in Boston, where his employers jealously kept him on short tether.

Dr. Farlow hovered over *James* as the bibliosleuth prepared to sail for Europe in 1920, steered him through his passport and tickets, fussed about his shots and whether he would make the boat in time, and whether he was spending too much or on the wrong books when he arrived. While her husband was abroad Mrs. Ballard confided on March 20 to the Librarian (and to his *Notes*) that "Jas. was very fond of dancing & had given lessons in Milton & had looked after dances in Odd Fellows Hall in Boston." There is no doubt that Ballard was a favorite with the ladies.

Each spring Jim Ballard embarked on a ritual visitation to the three larger medical libraries in New York, Philadelphia and Washington, repairing fences, buying, selling, exchanging, and enlarging his own reputation for an almost mythical astuteness. In 1920 he turned down the offer of the assistant librarianship of the Philadelphia College of Physicians (with promise of the top job in time), because the money wasn't good enough, and in 1921 rejected the associate editorship of the *Index Medicus* in Washington. And yet he remained unsure enough of himself and his position that he would accede to the most unjustified limitations imposed on his extracurricular life by his bosses, who apparently were afraid that professional honors and offers might turn his head or coax him away. "Told James members of the exec. comm. were not in favor of his being candidate for president of the Med. Lib. Assoc.," Farlow wrote in his *Notes* on April 21, 1925. And on May 17, 1926: "Asked Ballard to withdraw as cand. for Treas. of Special Libraries Assn, as Ex. C. didn't favor his taking it."

While the assistant librarian early in his career was schooling himself in medical bibliography, especially incunabula, writing occasional articles and preparing papers and exhibits for the Boston Medical History Club, his singular contribution to library science was organizational. Blank slate that he was (like the old soldiers John Shaw Billings made experts of), he intuitively apprehended the elements of the first rough attempts at systematization of the medical literature under the tutelage of Dr. Chadwick and Mrs. Collins. He first described the Library's unique classification in January 1918 in the *Bulletin of the Medical Library Association*. In November of 1919 General Robert E. Noble and Colonel Fielding H. Garrison visited 8 The Fenway to see what features might be incorporated in the new Surgeon General's Library then being contemplated; they decided to adopt the Boston classification as propounded by Ballard.

Interest in the Boston system prompted publication—this time by the Library itself in 1925—of a second, enlarged edition of *The Boston Medical Library Medical Classification*, with a foreword by Ballard explaining that the scheme in use in 1879 had been revamped by Dr. Chadwick and Mrs. Collins on the *Index Medicus* pattern, but modified by bringing under one heading all material of a special nature. Thus everything cardiac was under *heart*, as opposed to the *Index*, which parceled it amongst anatomy, surgery, physiology and so on. The Boston system was simpler and more logical, Ballard wrote, and "particularly lends itself to congested conditions, which are not uncommon in medical libraries." By this time the BML Classification had been adopted by the Medical Library Association as the standard (in 1921) and by a growing number of institutions, including the library of the Harvard Medical School. When the second edition appeared, a fellow librarian

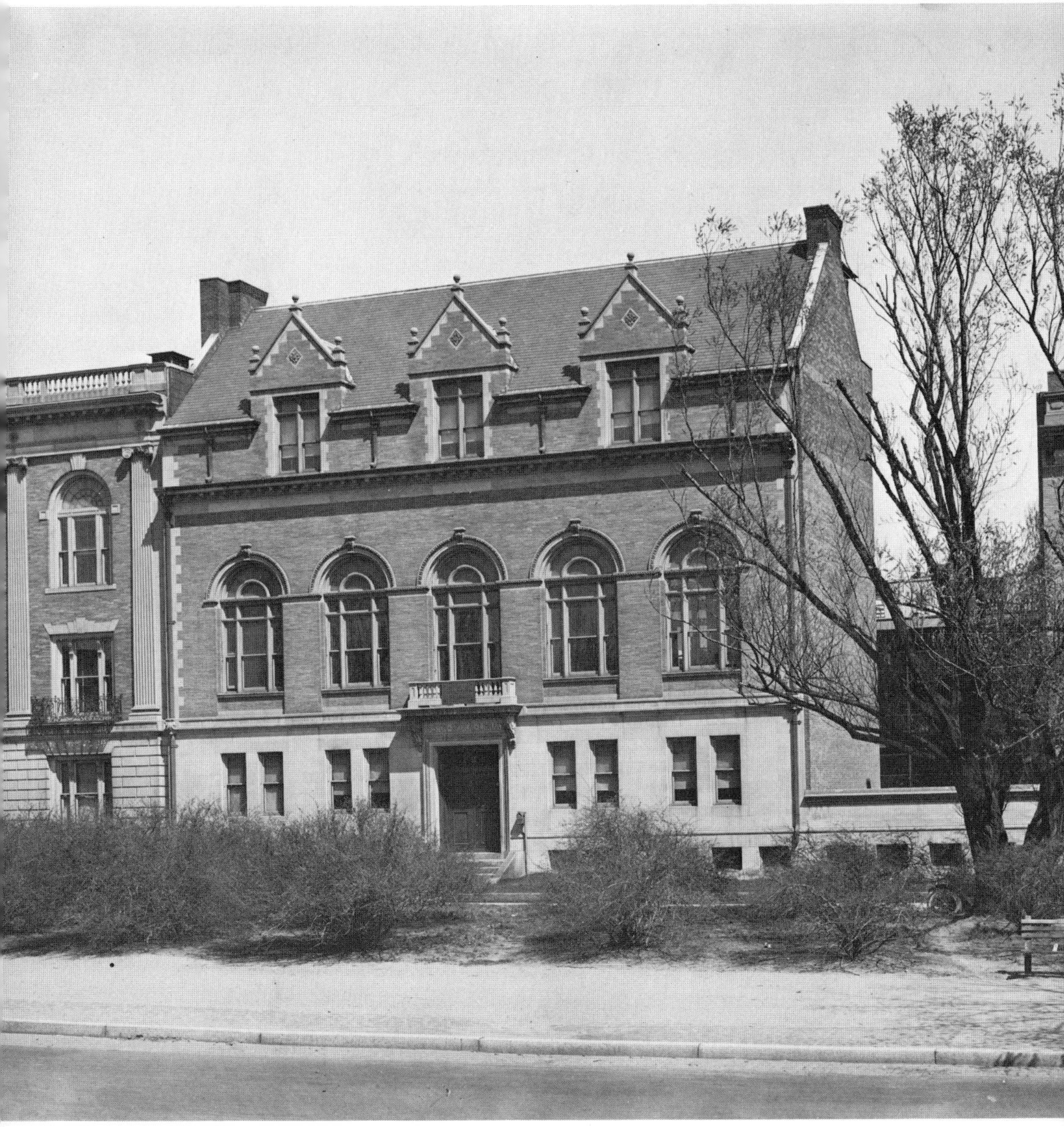

8 The Fenway, 1919

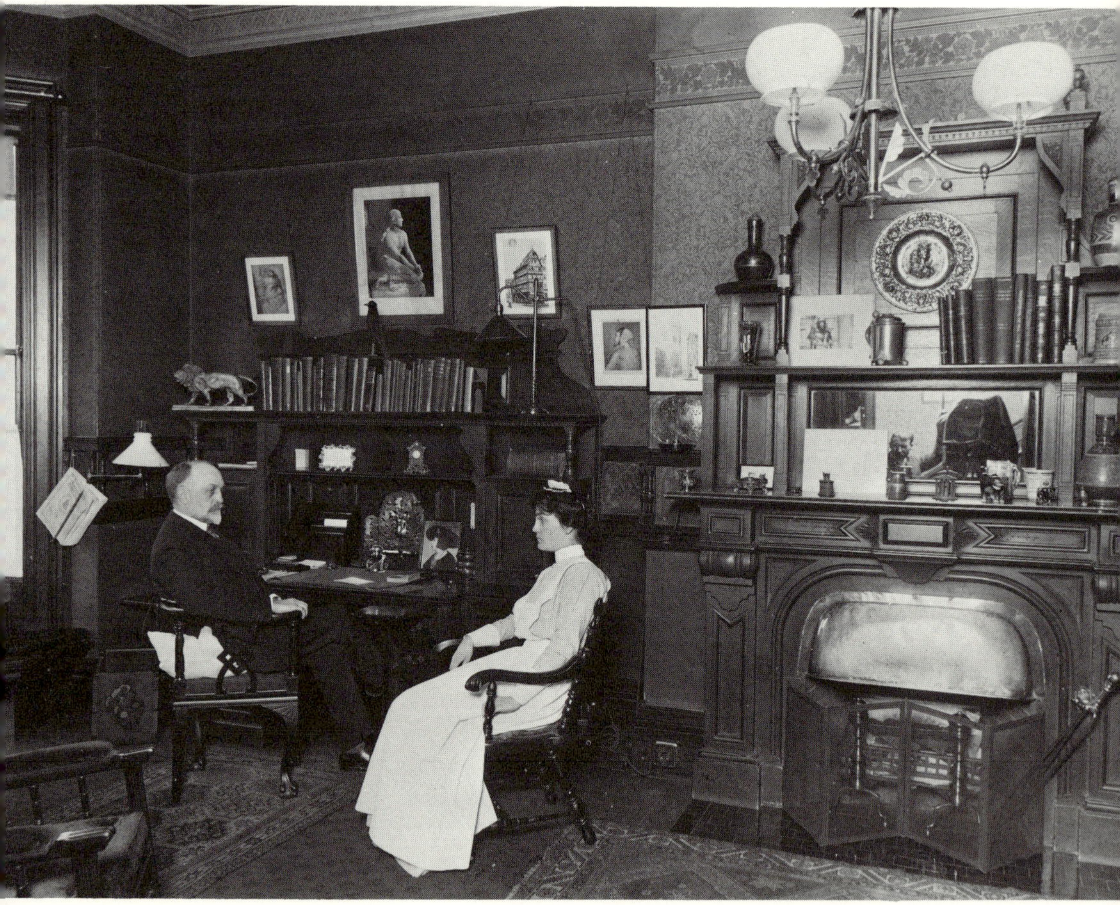

John W. Farlow, M.D., the second Librarian, in his medical office with his nurse at 234 Clarendon Street, 1914

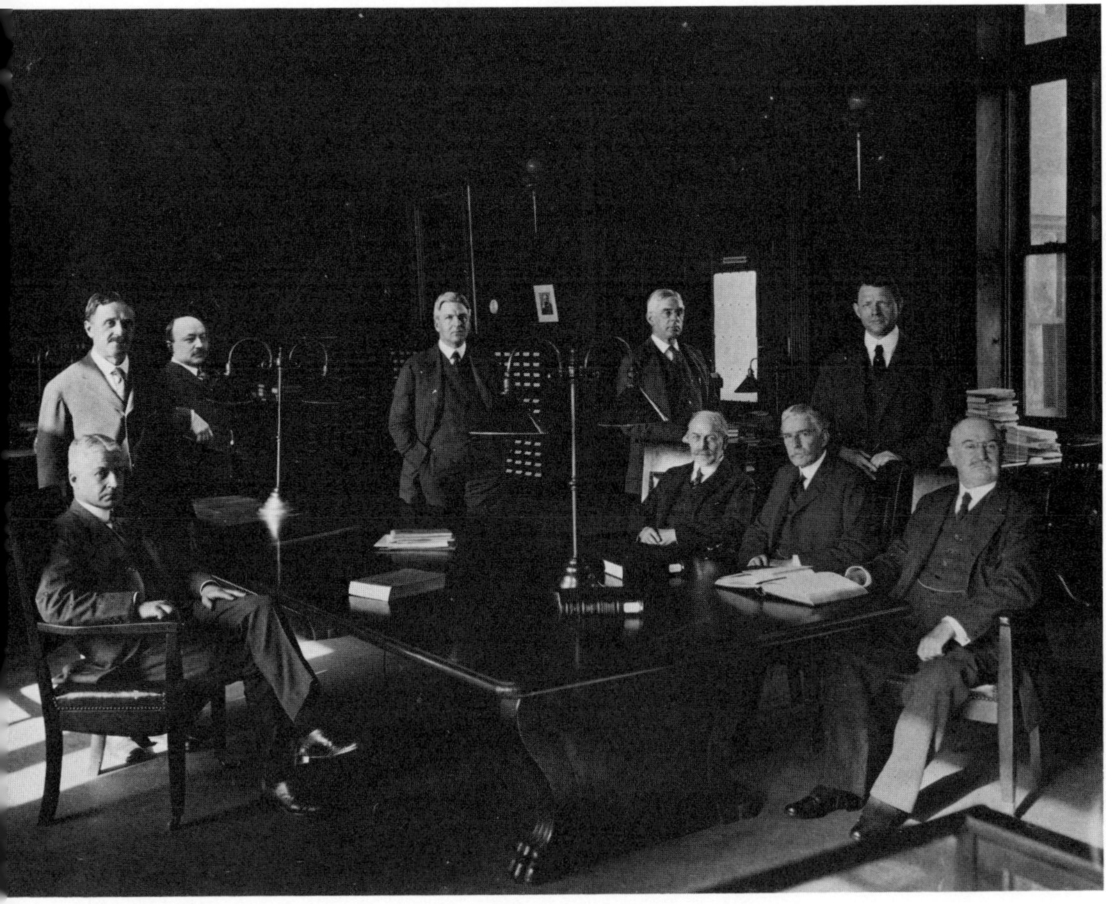

The Executive Committee, June 1921. Sitting, left to right, Richard G. Wadsworth, M.D., John W. Farlow, M.D., George H. Monks, M.D., and Walter L. Burrage, M.D.; standing, John W. Cummin, M.D., Malcom Storer, M.D., Edward C. Streeter, M.D., John W. Bartol, M.D., and Stephen Rushmore, M.D. Dr. Storer, who was not present, was pasted in by the photographer as if standing, from another picture of him sitting.

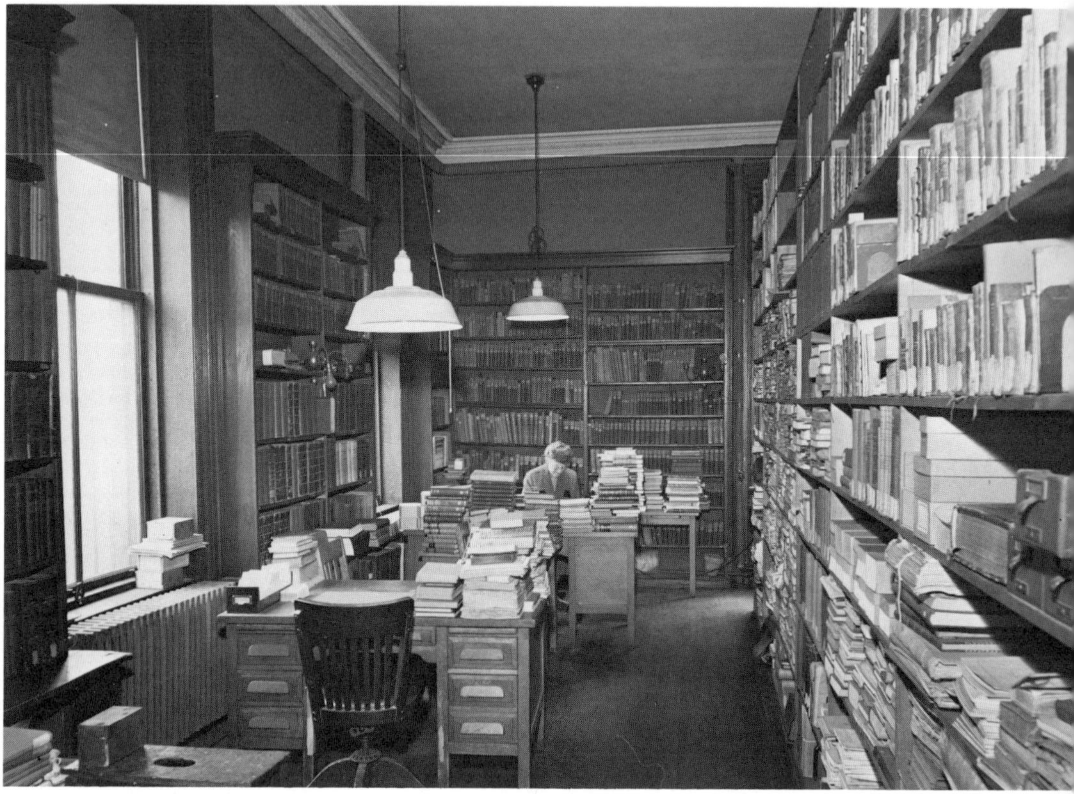

Catalogue Room, 8 The Fenway, Mrs. Ella F. Crosby at desk

James F. Ballard, about 1953

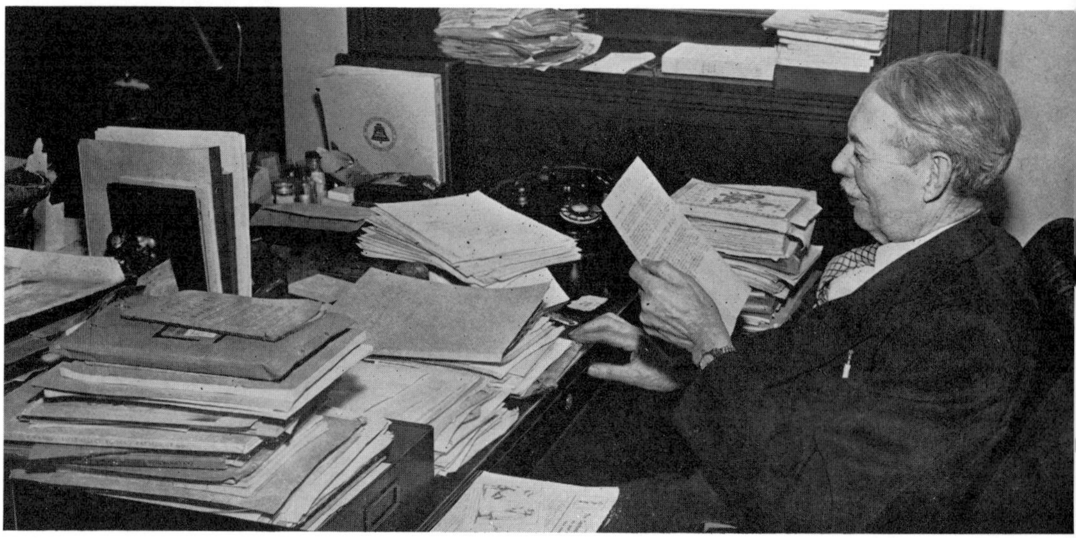

wrote some years later with a vestige of resentment which he could not conceal, "a strong protest was voiced at the Annual Meeting over the fact that it had been published by the Library rather than by the Association. Mr. Ballard defended the Library's publication of it, and no action was taken. . . Wide adoption of the classification here and abroad, of course did much to extend Mr. Ballard's reputation and that of his Library."[13]

After twenty years on the shelf, the academy of medicine proposition was taken down and dusted off again in 1924. This time the initiative came from Dr. Walter Bowers, the first editor of the still vagrant *Boston Medical and Surgical Journal* under the ownership of the Massachusetts Medical Society over which he had presided a decade earlier. Dr. Bowers was in general practice in the western town of Clinton, knew well the isolation of physicians who had not the advantage of academic affiliation close at hand, and he was in a special position, owing to the universal esteem in which he was held, to mount an effort to bridge these voids. And he badly needed proper editorial offices for the *Journal*. In November Bowers invited interested parties to consider the creation of what he called (not in the clinical sense) a *medical center*.

The executive committee of the Boston Medical Library, having but recently freed itself of the predatory embrace of Harvard, examined this proposition at a good arm's length, wondering whether to stand pat and try to finish off the stack wing, whether to move somewhere else, or whether to do anything at all, and voted in December to wait and see what kind of an offer was made.

Early in 1925 a special subcommittee of the Bowers committee sounded out the BML on the idea of a revived academy of medicine. The chairman was Channing Frothingham, one of the young organizers of the Brigham in 1912, a crescendo voice in the counsels of the Harvard Medical School, a social liberal destined gleefully to infuriate the organized profession with his advocacy of compulsory health insurance, a Brooklyn native, and a wit who is said to have replied to his father's query whether he had learned anything as a Harvard undergraduate: "Three things—to drink a fair amount of whiskey, to play a fair game of poker, and not to go back to Brooklyn."[14]

At a joint meeting with the executive committee on January 23, 1925 Dr. Frothingham described the need for a central gathering place for physicians who were unconnected academically, possibly along the lines of the projected expansion of the New York Academy of Medicine, yet too ambitious in scope for any accommodation at 8 The Fenway; if the response was affirmative, his group would recommend to the full

Bowers committee to apply to the Carnegie Corporation or Rockefeller Foundation for support, contingent on the support of the Medical Library.

In the view of Dr. Farlow and Dr. John W. Bartol of the executive committee, the BML had served effectively as an academy since the concept was broached at the turn of the century. The Librarian was characteristically emphatic in stating that if only the funds could be found to finish the addition, ample space would be reserved therein for both the *Journal* and the Medical Society.

Through the spring and summer of 1925, as inflation bore into the budget of the Library and hard money tightened, the Frothingham committee dreamed on. In October it presented plans for an academy of medicine at the southeast corner of Brookline and Longwood avenues which so impressed the executive committee that it voted on the spot to move the Library there if and when the money could be raised. It was not until the howls of dissent were heard above the winds of winter that the officers began reconsidering their euphoric endorsement. One such premonitory rumbling had already been recorded in his *Notes* by Dr. Farlow on September 15, via Ballard, who had inquired of Dr. William Norton Bullard, a vice president and the Library's well-endowed patron of incunabula, what he thought of the medical center notion; growled Bullard to Ballard, "those people would not get a cent of *his* money."

The fiftieth anniversary of the Boston Medical Library was observed sedately under the glowering dragons of John Ware Hall at the annual meeting on January 19, 1926. In April the executive committee again faced a fork in the way: the Academy of Medicine had actually been incorporated, with Frothingham as clerk, and the Library was under pressure to join. Their loyalties rewarmed in the afterglow of that golden jubilee, the officers held aloof, arguing the vagueness of the Academy's plans, the dubious advantages to the Library, their hopes of a financial bonanza. The occasion was chosen by Dr. Burrage to announce that the increasing strain put on his useless legs by attendance at the monthly meetings compelled his resignation as secretary, a position he had filled with honor for fifteen years. He was succeeded by Dr. Horace Binney, HMS 1901, a surgeon and a booklover.

In May the paper Academy sent forth a subcommittee under the persuasive Dr. Roger I. Lee, who repeated the complimentary admonition that the foundations could not be approached until the Library's cooperation had been secured. Both he and Frothingham pledged the autonomy of the BML within the Academy, and its freedom to withdraw at any time. The executive committee decided not to join for yet a while, but said it was still interested. The legal opinion of Henry L. Shattuck was sought; in December he advised that he did not believe the Library could lawfully participate under the existing constitution and by-laws of the Academy, and the officers bowed to his judgment with some relief.

Dr. Monks resigned unexpectedly as president in March 1927, within a few days of his seventy-fourth birthday and less than a year after his retirement as professor of oral surgery at the Harvard Dental School. The executive committee elected one of its own, John Washburn Bartol, to fill his unexpired term. Dr. Bartol was sixty-three, a native of Lancaster, a graduate of Harvard College and the Medical School (1891), where he was an assistant in clinical medicine from 1899 to 1909, a physician, a vice president of the Library from 1914 to 1920, and president of the Massachusetts Medical Society from 1921 to 1923. His election was affirmation of the close relationship with the Society, two of whose presidents, Cheever and Shattuck, were his predecessors in office at the Library, and whose librarian from 1884 until 1922 was Dr. Brigham, the genial and devoted host of the BML from its founding, who died on September 14, 1926 at eighty-six.

The legal obstacles to partnership in the Academy of Medicine aside, there remained the ever-tighter space squeeze upon the BML, and the longing of the Medical Society for quarters ample enough under one roof for its own expanding functions and for its *Journal*. These considerations weighed so heavily with the executive committee that in May 1927 it rejected an architect's plan for an expansion and endowment program that together would cost $350,000, the consensus being that the projected usefulness of forty years was insufficient, and space allocated to the Society and *Journal* inadequate. The alternative of a fresh start in a new location was again debated. "Much hot air. No progress," sniffed Dr. Farlow.[15]

The mounting demands and strains put upon the Library as it began its second half-century give pause when it is recalled that the last new shelf space, the 1909 basement stack addition, was overflowing by 1910 when the book census was about 70,000; yet by the end of 1927, somewhere had been shoehorned 75,000 more, a full doubling to 145,000 volumes and 96,000 pamphlets. Such were the peaks of the range, rising behind the foothills of the uncatalogued, those *basses Alpes* of the basement whose mass that year had so depressed the floors that it was necessary to excavate and remove truckloads of them to a storage warehouse.

To catalogue was to count the grains in a sand pile. The staff calculated that it completed 20,016 cards in 1927. The last of 30,000 German dissertations purchased sixteen years earlier was authored, titled, classified and numbered, but another 20,000 German and French theses begged regimentation, and the Kobert library on pharmacology and toxicology remained unappreciated in its packing boxes after four years. Each day the file of 742 current periodicals spun off its quota of back issues. The great entrance doors facing the park groaned grudgingly ajar to 10,035 users of 26,752 books and journals and 2695 attenders of fifty-four meetings of fifteen societies.

The litany of tabulation became a wearisome round to one who had recited it annually for a score of years, always in a minor key ("stacks that were overcrowded a year ago are getting into a condition where satisfactory work is next to impossible, and our patient catalogers and librarians are sorely tried to know how to deal with a problem which seems impossible of solution."). During the summer of 1927 Dr. Farlow made up his mind to retire at the end of the year. He notified President Bartol on September 5, a week after his seventy-fourth birthday. By mid-November his successor had been selected and agreed to serve, Charles Fairbank Painter, a member of the executive committee and the committee on the library, long active in its affairs.

Dr. Painter was Michigan-born on May 19, 1869, an early graduate of Johns Hopkins University, then of Harvard Medical School in 1895 with Elliott Joslin and Harvey Cushing, who wrote of his new friend to his father in their first year: "Painter I like very much. He is slow, but hangs on to everything he gets. He hails from Great Barrington, Mass. and is a great big solid whole-souled creature such as one likes to meet."[16] Painter and Cushing trained at the MGH, where the whole-souled creature came under the influence of Edward H. Bradford and Robert W. Lovett, pioneers in orthopedics, who steered him into their specialty. For years he was surgeon-in-chief at the Carney Hospital, briefly editor of *The Journal of Bone and Joint Surgery* and president of the American Orthopedic Association in 1915-1916. Behind the busy surgeon was the educator and the scholar. From 1913 to 1922 Painter was Dean of the Tufts Medical School, where his interests in literature and medical history led to the creation of the professorship of the history of medicine, which he held for some years.

During the lame-duck tenure of Dr. Farlow at the end of 1927 President Emeritus Monks organized a New England physicians' art exhibit at the Library which attracted three hundred avocational productions ranging from paintings to ship models, violins, and the most extraordinary minutes of the old Dorchester Medical Club kept by the late Dr. C.

Ellery Stedman and illustrated with his amusing and frequently ribald cartoons. On the final day, December 14, Dr. Farlow heard from President Bartol that there had been some comment about the Stedman notebook, that it was displayed "in spite of its being rather 'shady' in places & should be excluded." Next day Farlow "looked at Stedman book, but exhib. closed last evening & it can do no further harm. I didn't see anything very wicked on a casual examination."[17]

A fortnight after the art show closed Dr. Monks had no great difficulty persuading Dr. Farlow to be portrayed by Marie Page. The sittings extended through the annual meeting on January 17, 1928, when the retiring Librarian presented his final report: "A medical library, no matter how much educational value it has. . . has not the general appeal that charitable institutions, such as hospitals and dispensaries, have; but the grave situation that now confronts us is one in which the general public should be willing to do their part in return for the opportunity generously and freely offered by us to avail themselves of our rich resources."[18]

President Bartol spoke warmly of him: "Our sensations of grief at the passing from active service of the officer of the Library who has done more than seemed possible for any one person to do are too acute to go into. . . We hope he will maintain a close association with the Library and will comment on the steps which will be taken in years to come."[19]

This the Emeritus did, beginning that evening in his *Notes*: "Rising vote of thanks for my service. . . Beer?, crackers & cheese after meeting." Three more weeks, on February 9: "My portrait hung in Holmes Hall over card catalog. Not easy to see in some lights. Best seen from between 2 long tables."

James Ballard had grasped the changing of the guard as an opportunity to suggest to Dr. Farlow that his title be upgraded from assistant librarian to Director, a nominal promotion which, with an enlargement of the executive committee by two members, was accomplished by amending the by-laws at the 1928 annual meeting after Dr. Bartol explained that Ballard had been serving in the directorial capacity anyway. "No change is made in his duties. We simply dignify the office by the title and leave it in good hands."[20]

One more, and basic, alteration in the Library's governance seemed important in order to gird it for a renewed try at the parapets of surplus capital, by assault or suit. "It has outgrown the building to a point of desperation," declared Dr. Bartol, now President in his own right. "For the past few years many projects have been considered and discussed and it has become imperative that the Library should extend the scope of its activities in order to enlarge the institution."[21] The first step was completed that April of 1928, when the General Court amended the charter by adding to the definition of purpose ("to establish and maintain a Library of Medicine and the Allied Sciences") the words *and the promotion and advancement of medical science and medical education.*

The second step was the culmination in October of a series of spring and summer sessions with committees of the Medical Society and the still-viable Academy of Medicine, when the executive committee voted to participate in a joint fund committee under the chairmanship of Dr. Roger Lee. This would be another effort—on a rising stock market—to raise the money to complete the addition for stacks and for offices for the Society and its official organ, which had just been renamed *The New England Journal of Medicine*.

They called it the United Building and Endowment Fund Campaign and hired the Fiscal Service Corporation to run it. The goal was $300,000 to build nine floors of new stacks onto the next-door basement, projected to absorb thirty-five years of growth, with offices for the Medical Society and the *Journal*; repairs and improvements to 8 The Fenway, $50,000; Library endowment, $150,000; Society endowment, $100,000; and endowment for the "medical center program" (the Academy of Medicine was not specifically mentioned in the campaign brochure, *The Doctor Calls the Patient*), $50,000. In all, $650,000.

Twelve months after the first call the stock market crashed down upon doctor and patient, as the Great War had on that earlier attempt, demonstrating again that physicians are no more psychic at economic and political prognosis than economists, politicians, stockbrokers and shopgirls. . . and as prone to diagnostic error. In the middle of December, Scudder, Stevens and Clark expressed confidence in the Library's investments after what they called the "recent fall in values;" as of their November 1 appraisal, the portfolio had depreciated only about ten per cent since 1928, and the brokerage felt justified in predicting that current income would exceed the previous year's by approximately $2000 (it did, actually, by $1651). By January 15, 1930, the extent of the shambles had still not been comprehended, and Librarian Painter was reassuring his members in his second annual report that "whereas it is more or less disheartening to attempt to administer a trust like a great Library devoted to the uses of an important profession in the face of adverse conditions, nevertheless we are very forunate here in that the excellent work which has been done in the past has prepared the Institution to stand up under the strain." He then went on to remonstrate that "the raising of funds for the purpose of a Medical Library is made difficult because the profession and the public alike are strangely indifferent to the relation that such an institution bears to the work the doctor has in hand and the significance of that work to the public health. If physicians were more alive to the value of the material which is at their service here it would be far more easy to show a supporting public wherein they owe a debt to the Library."[22]

Two not indifferent to the purpose of medical libraries were Harvey Cushing, who at the beginning of 1930 faced in two more years the compulsory retirement which he had insisted on as a policy of the Brigham, and his admired old preceptor from Baltimore days, the pathologist and shaper of Johns Hopkins Medical School with Osler and Halstead, William H. Welch, for whom Hopkins had named its own medical bibliotheca in 1929. A couple of months before his eightieth birthday, in February of 1930, "Popsy" Welch, a born bachelor, entrained for Boston to help the Medical Library's bogged-down fund drive, and Dr. Cushing wrote an amused account of his arrival:[23]

> They had been trying without success to raise money in Boston to renovate and increase the stack-room in the Boston Medical Library. Quinby [Dr. William C. Quinby], who was on the Committee, dropped into my dressing room one morning and said he had run across Dr. Welch at a meeting somewhere and the idea occurred to him that possibly Dr. Welch might be persuaded to come on and give a talk about medical libraries and their purposes. This would draw a crowd and possibly increase the number of contributions. Dr. Welch said of course he would be glad to come.
>
> To ask an outside physician to come and help the Boston profession out of their financial difficulties was bad enough, but Dr. Welch of all people with his 80th birthday in the offing and the date set for the meeting in midwinter. "You don't for a moment expect that even if he meant it he will remember to come or remember what other engagements he may have made for the same evening," I remarked. "Oh yes," said Quinby confidently, "I saw him write it down in his little book." "What arrangements are you going to make for him?" I asked. "That's where you come in," he replied. "Can't you put him up?" So I wrote, knowing that he always preferred to go to a hotel rather than a private home, and he promptly accepted. It is just possible, as he hints in the note that soon followed, his real motive in accepting was to give the Boston Library a good looking over in preparation for what was soon coming in Baltimore.

Dr. Cushing and his chauffeur met Dr. Welch at the Back Bay railroad station early in the slushy morning of February 5 and brought him to his Brookline home for breakfast. The visitor had a number of friends he wanted to see, and his host told Popsy he could have the car after he had been dropped off at the Brigham. As they were leaving, the surgeon noticed a rash of spots, apparently of food, on the Welch waistcoat. They defied all the efforts of the household to exorcise them. And so a stop was made at a tailor's en route to the Brigham:

We meanwhile sat in the window at Bergstein's in Brookline Village while the deed was accomplished, and Popsy remarked that we were extraordinarily particular people here in Boston about our guests and their appearance—that he had bought this suit in Paris only eighteen months ago and he didn't see why it wasn't good enough for Boston. . . After all, the aim of this recital was not to point out Popsy's indifference to his personal appearance, for he was naturally tidy. It was rather to emphasize his disregard of himself in coming to Boston in midwinter at eighty years of age to make a speech in behalf of the Boston Library and to help it to raise some funds.

The plans of the Boston Medical Library to entrench itself more firmly than ever on the Fenway rekindled, in a brief flareup, that missionary flame in the breast of Professor Frederic T. Lewis. Dr. Lewis's zeal for a "medical Widener" somewhere between Shattuck Street and Longwood Avenue had not been assuaged by the reorganization and expansion of the Harvard Medical School library which Dean Edsall had implemented in 1928 with $200,000 obtained to enhance its usefulness to the School of Public Health. By converting the old lecture room in the administration building to stacks and making various other alterations that added to the reading room, the shelf space had been increased nearly threefold, hopefully enough to contain growth for another twenty or more years. In a decade the School library budget had increased from $3480 to more than $18,000, the number of volumes from 33,000 to 48,500, and pamphlets from 58,500 to 112,200, while through curricular reforms allowing students more free time, annual visits had risen from 13,150 to 34,600, and circulation from 4000 to 21,500. Dr. Edsall was proud of these statistics, remarking that "an adequate library is so near to being the heart of the activities of the students and the staff. . ."[24]

But still neither adequate nor hearty enough for Professor Lewis, who selected the second of May, 1930, to resume his long-dormant campaign to persuade President Lowell that the University ought to commit itself to a great new medical library of its own. It could have been no secret among the faculty that the next day Edsall was to take for his third wife his secretary, Louisa Richardson, and then to sail for Europe immediately on a wedding trip of four months. The Dean would be on the high seas when the President opened the Professor's letter:

I am well aware that the Dean has no adequate appreciation of the importance to the School of its library, or he would have found some way out of our predicament, difficult though the way may be. . . There can be no first class medical school without a library to correspond; and Harvard's situation is evident when one reflects that if Dr. Cushing were to remain as Harvard's Dr. Welch, there would be no library for him to preside over. . . Johns Hopkins now has 50,000 volumes; the Boston Medical Library has 150,000. Under expert guidance of Garrison[25] and with resources, they will fill their empty stacks. But if Harvard could secure what Harvard men, as members of the Boston Medical Library have gathered, there would be nothing to envy at Johns Hopkins in this respect.[26]

President Lowell was firmly loyal to his absent Dean and responded noncommittally that it was as unlikely as ever that the Medical Library would move near the School, and furthermore: "It is surely unwise for the Harvard Medical School to try to duplicate the Medical Library in old books that are of use chiefly for historical purposes, and which are rare and expensive. I agree that the School ought to have the use—like all parts of the University—of the largest possible collection of books and periodicals; but, on the other hand, these things ought not to be needlessly duplicated within a mile of each other."[27]

Professor Lewis next tackled Worth Hale, Acting Dean in Edsall's absence, urging him to lobby with the powers in the Medical School and University to make a final effort at enticing the Medical Library to join the School in a well-endowed new building. . . "and I think that to set them going in the absence of the big chief is your opportunity. At least a full realization of just what is being done to the School by enlarging the library in the Fenway should be made known. . ."[28]

In a guarded reply to this unguarded blandishment, Dr. Hale allowed that he had already initiated some inquiries on his own and was not sanguine. "If anything can be accomplished I imagine a certain amount of diplomacy will be necessary and I also think it would take a very considerable amount of money, in any case, and I do not know now where we might secure it."[29]

Scattering his shots, Lewis in the same mail begged Harvey Cushing to spurn the rumored advances from Hopkins and remain in Boston after his retirement to build up the Harvard library. Perhaps wings could be grafted on Building A, enlarging the library into a medical Widener of a size to attract the rival on the Fenway. "A major and blighting defect" in the honeymooning Edsall's administration, he wrote Cushing, was "his failure to appreciate our library situation." Lewis had visited the new Hopkins library named for Welch and returned to Boston, "thinking of the dean's complacent report [at a recent faculty meeting] on the increase in the use of our books, and the growth of our library from a little to a small one."[30]

Harvey Cushing's battles with David Edsall off and on for a dozen years over policy, purse and personality were proverbial, and he replied:[31]

Dear Fred:

I got your letter Saturday with the exchange of letters with Mr. Lowell. I tried to get in touch with you, hoping that I might talk things over with you; but I found you had gone, for which I was glad rather than disappointed as I liked to think you were taking advantage of a beautiful day to get in the open.

Now I subscribe to everything you say about the Library and the Dean's neglect of it. Unfortunately he is not built on classical lines, and I don't think he has much interest in books or appreciates what they mean. If he could wangle $25,000 out of the Foundation to pay for that humiliating "Synopsis of the Practice of Preventive Medicine," what might he not have wangled out of them to bring the Boston Medical Library up to our neighborhood? But then, we'll have to gulp this down with whatever wry face we must make in the effort.[32]

So far as making any change at present in the plans of the Boston Medical Library, I think it is too late. The authorities are wedded to the idea of staying where they are, and so stay they will, I judge, until you and I have passed on. If I were younger and as energetic as I was when I first came here, I would have struggled to do what I personally could toward bringing the Library here. But my single small contribution to our own library consisted in struggling for such fusion of the departmental libraries as now exists, and I shall have to let it go at that.

Possibly when 1932 comes around and for the first time in many years I shall have a little freedom, I might be willing to tackle the problem anew. It is quite possible, indeed probable so far as I can gather, that the sum which the Library is hoping to raise may not be secured. If that is so, we could then perhaps persuade the B.M.L. Association to move out in this neighborhood.

All this talk about my going to Baltimore to step into Popsy's boots began, I think, more or less as a jest; at least I have never taken it very seriously and Welch is good for another ten years. You will remember what Edison said when some news gatherer asked him when he was going to retire and he ejaculated: "Retire! Never! It's unhealthy." I hope and believe that Popsy is imbued with the same spirit.

Always affectionately yours,
Harv Cushing

Cushing was only forty per cent correct in his prediction of the longevity of Welch (who died on April 30, 1934), and he shifted not to Hopkins but to Yale, as Sterling Professor of Neurology in 1932, all in spite of Edsall's efforts to keep him at Harvard. And to Yale he bequeathed his superb personal medical library, thereby fulfilling an early foreboding on that account which cropped up in Dr. Farlow's *Notes* in 1927: "Feb. 26. Dr Harvey Cushing thinks we are trying to get too many collections turned over to us. James has been told that Dr. C. is going to give his books to Yale."

Dr. Cushing was on the mark in his assumption that the fund drive for the enlargement of the Boston Medical Library would fall short. It did, unhappily, as the early stages of the Great Depression gripped the land, but not short enough to dissuade the members of the executive committee—even as Professor Lewis, in all ignorance of their action, was counteragitating—from a decision to go ahead with what they had (eventually about $240,000 when the books of the United Building and

Endowment Fund were finally closed), which was $100,000 less than was needed to build the raison d'être of the entire project, the stacks themselves.

By the end of 1930 the shell of the addition, hard against Number 22, the former Peabody residence, and facaded to match Number 8, was roofed over and heated. The old headquarters of the Directory of Nurses were made over into staff offices in memory of the first secretary, Dr. Oliver F. Wadsworth, by his family. The former Chadwick Periodical Room on the third floor of the old building was refitted by the widow of Dr. Morton Prince in his memory as a reading room containing his private library, and current journals were moved to the second floor, between Holmes Hall and the new building.[33] *The Journal of Bone and Joint Surgery*, hallmarked by its familiar *os* nailed to the door, moved into the former "Supper Room" in July of 1931.

That September the Massachusetts Medical Society and *The New England Journal of Medicine*, organically anastomosed at last, occupied the addition. Above them was space, seven gaping, floorless levels of it, as empty of stacks and books as were the hopes of the dreamers for filling it.

9

Doldrums

1930 · 1941

> Water, Water, everywhere,
> And all the boards did shrink.
> *The Ancient Mariner*

In the track of Coleridge's fated ship, the Boston Medical Library drifted through the doldrums of the Great Depression on an undrinkable sea of special funds, entailed, bound, and forbidden for the maintenance of life. On deck the level in the meagre casks of unrestricted income, though short-rationed, dropped by the day, causing the crew some intervals of thirst less than slaked, though fortunately no black lips baked.

By 1934 the Library was skimming off capital to pay debts; book purchasing was curtailed, periodicals cancelled, back issues left unbound; maintenance declined; members fell away; dues were forgotten; the reference librarian was cast adrift; the remaining crew were obliged to take a ten per cent pay cut; and an operating deficit of $1346 was entered in the log.

> Water, water, everywhere,
> Nor any drop to drink.

At the end of 1934 the treasurer had grimly to report a surplus of $18,000 of income from restricted funds, unspent for lack of anything to spend it on, banned by the strictures of gifts and bequests from deployment against general expenses. The whole endowment was divided between unrestricted funds with a book value of $108,000, and $214,789 in restricted investments; their combined market worth was only about $275,000.

This two-to-one disproportion of designated to free income had its most penurious effect on the periodical file. Less than $1000 in annual restricted income was reserved for journals, against upwards of $6000 required. This benign neglect of the serial literature by benefactors had given rise years before the Crash to the pernicious practice of compensatory borrowing from special income, a picking of the Petrian pocket which by 1933 had contributed $18,000 to a Paullist deficit of $30,000. These well-intentioned and perhaps unavoidable misappropriations did not diminish over the years as a chronic source of budgetary embarrassment. As it turned out, the stratagem staved off the evil day until a more acceptable subterfuge could be devised, and it certainly palliated the pain if not the process of depression. The single staff casualty was the reference librarian who had been taken on in 1928 to assist members in their bibliographic searchings; she was let go in 1932 and not replaced. On June 1, 1933 the five remaining staff under Director Ballard accepted a ten per cent cut in pay, and the Library was closed evenings. Book purchases not specially funded were curtailed. During the worst of it some of the more expensive and expendable foreign journals were stopped, as well they might have been, considering that only four months after the panic, in February 1930, the executive committee approved the sale of securities to pay Otto Enslin, a German bookseller, $6500 owed for periodicals. Orders for binding were cut back; equally without excuse, the BML had fallen $7800 in arrears to U. Holzer, Inc., its Boston binder since the beginning, and it was only through the personal generosity of Dr. Farlow that $3000 of this was forwarded to his old friends in March of 1930.

The irony of the Depression with the sharpest edge was the bestowal of three restricted funds, bountiful in the aggregate, whereby the Library, though it was lopping off contemporary journals right and left, was compelled to gather one of the largest and most comprehensive collections of antiquarian medical works in existence.

It all germinated from two rare seeds buried within the personal library which Dr. Holmes had deposited at Boylston Place. . . his *Canon* of Avicenna, printed in 1490, and his *Aphorisms* of Maimonedes, 1489. These were joined by a first edition of the *Fasciculus medicinae* of Johannes de Ketham, 1491, the earliest printed medical book containing illustrations and the only copy in America, acquired at the Boston auction of the David Hunt collection in 1893 by Dr. John Homans 2nd while a member of the executive committee, and presented by him to the Library. These three were the first sprouts in the garden of incunabula and lesser varieties of nascent medical printing which awaited the spadework of William Norton Bullard and the cultivation of James Francis Ballard to bloom like desert blossoms (where all around was parched) in wonderful splendor.[1]

Dr. Bullard was a well-to-do Newporter, born five days ahead of his friend John Farlow, on August 23, 1853, but three years behind him at Harvard Medical School in the class of 1880, in consequence of a bout with typhoid fever. House pupilship at the MGH preceded a year in Vienna and concentration on neurology, his specialty on his return to Boston, where over the next score of years he was on the staffs of the Dispensary, City Hospital working with Morton Prince and Philip C. Knapp, the Carney and Children's hospitals, and the State Hospital for Epileptics at Palmer, of which he was a founder and a chairman of the trustees. He published widely and achieved international recognition early as a pioneer in neurology, retiring from active practice in 1902 and gradually from his professional associations because of poor health. In 1909 he endowed the William Norton Bullard Professorship of Neuropathology at Harvard.

Precise, reserved, married but childless, Dr. Bullard collected wildflowers and the literature of neurology and historical medicine. His first official connection with the Boston Medical Library was in 1899 as a member of the committee to raise funds for the Fenway building. By 1907 he was donating volumes of rare periodicals in neurology and mental diseases. In 1910 he presented his first incunable, an event so unremarked on that Dr. Farlow in his annual report passed it off as "a copy of Arnoldus de Villa Nova, 1491," without benefit of title or further description.[2] For the next seven years Bullard collected sixteenth and seventeenth century texts, five of which he gave to the Library, as well as some works in medical botany, before adding his second fifteenth-century imprint to the collection, Johannes de Gaddesden's *Rosa anglica practica medicinae*, printed in 1492. That was in 1917; in 1918 he was elected a vice president.

By 1920, when he contributed four of them, the connoisseur was concentrating on incunabula, and beginning in 1926, exclusively so. Having then given fifteen in all to the BML, he decided to combine with these his own and in 1927 shelved the lot in Holmes Hall as the "William Norton Bullard Loan Collection of Medical Incunabula," made the subject of a nicely printed and hardbound catalogue compiled by Ballard and issued privately in 1929.[3] In the meanwhile Bullard had redoubled his collecting efforts in the face of heart disease and failing eyesight. In 1928 he added twenty-five incunabula to the loan collection and some five hundred sixteenth and seventeenth-century volumes to those already credited to him, in addition to a number of more recent works dealing with epilepsy. Thirty-one more incunables in 1929 swelled the aggregate to 182, those acquired by the Library from other sources to fifty-four. Still avidly combing the lists in 1930, the antiquarian bought another thirty-two, while the Library acquired six, raising the respective collections to 214 and sixty.

In his Introduction to the *Catalogue* Ballard outlined the objective of the Bullard Collection:

> The books have been collected with the definite idea of bringing together the works on medicine and related sciences which were printed in the fifteenth century. Particular attention has not been given to printers or presses and very little stress placed on first editions, except in a few instances. The medieval student's greatest need was dictionaries to interpret the new works flowing into the language from foreign sources. Medical terms and definitions are contained in most of the fifteenth century dictionaries and for this reason the Bullard Collection includes many examples of this class of book. The Arabian authors are very well represented, and the collection is also strong in the philosophical field of medicine as evidenced by the numerous texts of Albertus Magnus, Nider, Sabunde, and others, and of Aristotle and his various commentators. Of special interest are the pest tracts and the various works on witchcraft, demons, sorcery and divination.[4]

No doubt Bullard leaned on Ballard and others expert in the narrow field of his collecting to offset occasional miscalculations which affected his aesthetic if not his literary judgment. According to Mrs. Bullard's nephew, John P. Coolidge, Professor of Fine Arts at Harvard, Dr. Bullard's brother, Francis, a collector of prints, presented the Bullards with a work by Julio Campagnola which for the rest of their lives they insisted on calling "our Dürer" notwithstanding its manifest style and the patent signature of the artist. "I must say it was perfectly extraordinary," recalls Professor Coolidge. "I remember my uncle as a retiring person with an air of arrogance about him which was perhaps really shyness, and very, very elegant. But he had absolutely no visual sense."[5]

William Norton Bullard died suddenly at the Ritz Carlton Hotel in Boston on April 13, 1931 at seventy-seven. He bequeathed to John Coolidge *our Dürer*, and to the Boston Medical Library all his incunabula, the balance of his personal medical library, and the sum of $50,000, of which the income and up to half the principal were designated for the purchase of books and manuscripts antedating 1700. He made the Library's the third largest collection of medical incunabula in the western hemisphere. The imprint of his unschooled lay collaborator on this scholarly achievement drew the admiration of medical bibliophiles, and it would be stamped deeper as the work continued.[6]

The Bullard passion for "fifteeners," the expertise of Ballard, the stimulus of the Boston Medical History Club under the influence of Harvey Cushing, Edward Streeter and a bookish young Cushing disciple, Henry Rouse Viets, the predisposition of Librarian Painter, and probably the relative availability of easy money, all had combined to boom interest in the classical literature of medicine in the late Twenties and in the first post-Crash months of unreality. In point of time, Dr. Bullard's bequest was the last of the restricted funds for antiquarian purchase. The first was $5000 received under the will of Dr. John Warren, the fifth in that durable line, son of Dr. J. Collins Warren and Associate Professor of Anatomy at Harvard, who died on July 17, 1928, less than twelve months after the passing of his father, who had given the Library a mass of family historical material over the years; the income from the Warren Fund was reserved for the acquisition of books on medical history, emphasizing anatomy. The second in order of the major pools of money restricted for historical purposes, $25,000, was secured in 1930 on the initiative of President Bartol from the trustees of the Godfrey M. Hyams Fund, to establish the Solomon M. Hyams Collection of Hebraic Medical Liberature; half of the principal was to be used to fill out the Library's existing collection in this area with works of historical significance, preserving the rest as endowment for the purchase of current literature on the subject.

These funds together amounted to $80,000, a considerable "no trespassing area" in the BML's endowment, and it was the pleasure of a whimsical fate that they should have been launched on their special mission just as economic disaster overtook the world, and the world market for medico-literary rarities. The Library had been spending about $7000 annually on books, but in doleful 1932 the strictures of the Bullard and Hyams funds dictated bargain-hunting to the tune of another $8000, while during even more impecunious 1933, $17,726 in capital and income from these two funds alone reaped eighty incunabula and twenty early manuscripts. On Ballard's advice the executive committee appointed Lathrop C. Harper, a New York book dealer and incunabulist, "Library Adviser," and Dr. Painter commented that "the historical collection of the Library is becoming well known throughout the country and its riches are attracting scholars in many fields of knowledge."[7]

The hoard of incunabula, 274 at Dr. Bullard's death, had by the end of 1934 been more than doubled by bargain purchases with the Bullard and Hyams funds (and a few from the Warren legacy) to a total of 565. In 1935 half the principal in each of the major bequests remained, and henceforth they were held as endowment.

Lincoln Davis followed John Bartol as president in 1933, the bottom of the Depression. Just retired at sixty as chief of the East Surgical Service of the MGH, where he had started the climb as a house pupil, Dr. Davis was a man of "solid common sense and high character" in the estimation of Frederic A. Washburn, the Director.[8] The new president had trekked east from Worcester to Harvard College and the Medical School (1898), where he taught anatomy for eight years, then surgery on the eve of World War I, when as a lieutenant colonel he initially had charge of surgery in Base Hospital 6 which Colonel Washburn recruited from the Mass General; later he served with American forces in Italy. After the war he helped set up the tumor clinic at the MGH and entered gynecology. He had been a member of the executive committee of the BML since 1927. Its third secretary, incidentally—Horace Binney—was succeeded in 1934 by Dr. James M. Faulkner, Harvard Medical School graduate of 1924 and faculty member, and physician at City Hospital and the MGH.

One of the first acts of the Davis administration (intended possibly to dispel any fears that the Boston Medical Library had anything to fear but fear itself) was the purchase of a thousand wooden boxes, coffin-size, and in the aggregate capable of containing eighteen thousand books. In a not particularly convincing show of confidence that this was anything but a temporary holding operation until $100,000 could be found to fill the cavernous addition with permanent steel stacks, the boxes were piled upon their sides, eventually from the first floor to the roof itself and clear around the inside perimeter of what Dr. Davis called "that aching void," each higher gallery gained by a higher flight of precarious wooden stairs and catwalk. For the lack of an elevator in the empty well, the crates were hoisted or lowered away by a hand-hauled block and tackle.

The other major inaugural act of the new president came as an unpleasant surprise to some of his associates, gauging from the sequelae, or rather, the absence of them. The gist is contained in a letter from Dr. Reginald Fitz, son of the pathologist, to Professor Robert P. Blake, Director of the Harvard University Library, dated September 2, 1933, informing him that "a few weeks ago the Committee of the Library of the Medical School voted that an effort be made to withdraw from the Boston Medical Library our books now on deposit there. I had a game of golf with Dr. Lincoln Davis, President of the Medical Library, wherein I received a serious licking, but afterwards we had luncheon in a most friendly manner. Dr. Davis feels that the Medical Library has no claim on our books, thus disagreeing with his predecessors. He feels that the Library may be somewhat reluctant to turn back our books which have been there for so long a time but that they must come home if the University so desires. . ."[9]

Fitz's interest had been aroused by a note from Harvard College Librarian Alfred C. Potter calling his attention to the circumstances under which the collection was deposited thirty years earlier. Obligingly, Professor Blake lodged a formal request with the Medical Library.[10]

September 6, 1933.

Dear Dr. Davis:

As you are doubtless aware, in 1902-1903 the Harvard College Library transferred on deposit some 3750 volumes dealing with medical subjects to the Boston Medical Library. At the time when this transfer took place, the College Library had completely outgrown its quarters and was terribly pressed for room. As the years went by, the situation changed both for the Harvard College Library in its new and commodious quarters in Widener, and for the Medical School in its new buildings. Over the same period there has been a distinct growth of interest in the history of medicine not only on the part of physicians, but also among scholars in nonmedical fields who have found rich treasures and rare bits of knowledge in early medical books. It is clear, I think, from the correspondence on the matter, through which I have just gone, that their status as a deposit was definitely fixed at the time of the transfer. It goes without saying that we are profoundly grateful to your Society and to the staff of your Library for housing and caring for this valuable collection at a time when we had no space and were at our wits' end to know where to shelve the ever growing flood of new acquisitions. I am sure, likewise, that these books under the new conditions will be equally accessible to the members of your Society and we hope that they will continue to use them in the same manner as members of the University continually consult the rare volumes ensconced upon your shelves.

May I, therefore, as Director of the Harvard University Library, request that you take up with the governing body of the Boston Medical Library a formal request on my behalf that the volumes from the Harvard College Library, deposited with them in 1902-1903 and amounting to 3750 volumes, be sent over to the Library of the Harvard Medical School?

With many thanks, etc.
Robert P. Blake

It was sixteen months, however, before Dr. Painter announced to the annual meeting of January 15, 1935 that "recently the Harvard Library has asked that these books be reassembled and returned. Progress is being made in meeting this request."[11] Another seventeen months elapsed, and although some of the books had been brought together at the BML, "the technical details of the transfer," in the words of Dr. Davis, "have not yet been worked out, but Professor Blake or his representatives at the Widener and the Director of our Library are working on them." This was June 30, 1936.[12] On July 17 Director Ballard expressed to the executive committee his hope that the change of librarians at Harvard might obviate the return of all or even any of the books. (On the verge of retirement, Potter and Blake were replaced in 1937 by one man, Keyes D. Metcalf.) Three more years of dawdling, and the Librarian reported in March of 1939 that about half of the books had been sent over to Harvard, and the parties had agreed to let it go at that for a while.[13]

Each year of the deepening Depression the Boston Medical Library endured further debilitation of investment income, from $27,589 in 1930 down to $15,283 in 1934, when the treasurer's pen dipped and came up red for fourteen years running. Seven thousand dollars were removed from capital in 1934 to wipe out accumulated debts for books and periodicals; yet $7700 for binding remained in the debit side of the ledger. Dr. Farlow again stepped forward, with $2000 this time, to help bail out his old bailiwick. Several of the medical societies responded to an appeal for journal subsidies with another $2000, and the three medical schools continued small voluntary "rent" on behalf of their students. But members kept slipping away by resignation and default. From 866 in 1933, the roster dropped to 829 in '34, a $510 loss of that unrestricted income on which the bread and butter of the Library depended. Delinquencies now totalled $2000. By 1937 membership had dropped to 779. "We take pride in our medical schools," complained Dr. Painter, "we glory in our philanthropic organizations; our hospitals we are pleased to regard as second to none, but our Medical Library, which nurtures them all, some seem disposed to forget."[14] Actually the reed of the profession's support was not quite as thin as the doctor painted it. The highest dues remittance in the Thirties was $10,498 in 1930, the lowest $9525 in 1939, when late in the year the trend was reversed in spectacular fashion by the feat of Dr. Benjamin Castleman in signing up 124 new members, largely at the MGH where he was a young pathologist. Upon Dr. Faulkner's resignation as secretary a few weeks later, the master recruiter was his natural successor.

The death of Justice Oliver Wendell Holmes on March 6, 1935, two days before his ninety-fourth birthday, released the unrestricted contingent bequest of $25,000 left the Library by his sister, the daughter of the first president, Mrs. Amelia Holmes Sargent, forty-six years earlier. To Lincoln Davis it was "a veritable godsend,"[15] and seemed to bring on a minor reversal of the Library's fortunes. The rising deficit of $23,123 incurred by borrowing from restricted income was nearly halved by using $10,700 of this manna to extinguish old periodical binding debts. The next $5000 was committed to overdue renovation and repairs. The balance was combined with $7000 from the building fund to construct two tiers of steel stacks, with cubicles and studies, in that aching void adjoining Number 8, enough running feet of shelf to absorb nearly 30,000 volumes without leaving much of a hole in the pile.

That standing debt to restricted income reproached the trustees. They had the uncomfortable feeling that they had been caught with the goods, like boys dipping into the cookie jar, and while the application of the salve released by the passing of a great American conscience eased theirs by halving the burden upon it, every treasurer's report evoked a twinge.

In 1937 what appeared to be a respectable way out was found. At its March meeting, acting upon the advice of counsel, the board recorded its "well considered opinion that volumes of periodicals and serials may properly and shall be held to constitute 'books' in the broad meaning of the word." By this sophistical sleight of semantics the trustees instructed the treasurer that the cost of bound periodicals not provided for by restricted funds from that moment on should be charged to income from special funds designated for the purchase of new books in those fields. A further rationale from counsel, which is perhaps more acceptable in retrospect, held that administrative expenses which hitherto had been borne entirely out of unrestricted income could fairly be charged to restricted funds, pro rata and retroactively.

Of course something had to be done when water, water was everywhere, but nary a drop to drink.

A third saving, which would mount up handsomely in the long run, began with the offer in 1938 of Vice President Robert N. Nye, the editor of *The New England Journal of Medicine* who had succeeded Dr. Bowers, to donate annually about a hundred exchange periodicals (allowing cancellation of the duplicate subscriptions), as well as review copies of books in return for reviews. These various measures, above board and below, helped along by cash from unrestricted gifts and bequests, had reduced the obligation to unexpended restricted income to $5450 by 1940.

Although the Library would finish 1936 under the largest deficit of the Depression, $4618, the officers opened the year feeling flush with the Sargent money and restored the staff pay cuts of 1933. In the spirit of institutional reform which was sweeping the land they steered a revision of the by-laws through the annual meeting limiting their terms (all but the Librarian) and replacing the executive committee of indeterminate service with a board of twelve rotating trustees. Qualifications for membership had already been liberalized through amendments adopted in 1935, adding associate and non-resident categories to the class of professional, or institutional, members created in 1929. These reforms were intended to attract younger men, as Dr. Painter explained (and more dues), and "to do away with any implication of 'star chamber' methods in the selection of those upon whom must fall the responsibility of administering this trust."[16]

President Roosevelt's Emergency Relief Appropriation Act was passed by Congress in April 1935 and set up the Works Progress Administration to substitute federally paid work for direct relief. Within a year 3,400,000 of the unemployed were raking leaves, painting murals and much else in between, such as inventorying and evaluating the Library's old paintings toward the end of 1936, a project which inspired the Director with possibilities truly herculean in scope. They boiled down to two, which Ballard presented to the trustees in August 1937: the mobilization of WPA talent to compile a union shelf list encompassing all the medical and biological collections in Greater Boston; and cataloguing and shelf-listing the backlog at the BML. Both were approved by the trustees, and soon by WPA officials, and before the year was out work was under way on the "Union Catalogue of Medical and Biological Books in Libraries of Metropolitan Boston," to be maintained at the Boston Medical Library for the assistance of the public in finding works wherever they were shelved in the area.

These companion WPA projects continued for three and a half years until their suspension by the national emergency on June 30, 1941. The Union Catalogue by then had been nearly completed, but a periodical binding job—not yet started though the equipment had been moved in—had to be aborted. The accomplishments of the WPA's first three years were assessed by President Davis at the annual meeting in January 1941:[17]

> The mass of periodicals and serials accumulated during twenty years, piled high in the basement, was examined and sorted. Items wanted by the library were catalogued and filed, the remainder disposed of by exchange or sale. Over 397,000 items were examined, 25,000 added to the files, over forty tons of materials disposed of, and 19,000 periodical and serial titles checked for the new edition of the *Union List of Periodicals and Serials*. Three hundred and seventeen thousand dissertations and theses, as well as several thousand bound volumes, have been examined, catalogued and shelved. The catalogue in Holmes Hall, which was in a sad state of dilapidation, was renovated, cleaned and partly retyped. Nearly sixty-three thousand volumes were vacuum cleaned and dusted. This work is still going on. In spite of the imposing amount of work done, much still remains, and I cannot say truthfully that our basement has as yet been transformed into a model of orderliness.

The WPA workers figured they had sifted through one hundred tons of material. The entire operation had cost the taxpayers about $55,000 and was considered worth $75,000 to the BML, whose out-of-pocket expenses of $1100 had been more than offset by the sale of duplicates discovered during the upheaval.

Hardly was this vast bibliographic raking project of the WPA's under way when, on January 26, 1938, the trustees took the unprecedented action of unanimously censuring Director Ballard for having failed to report what was cryptically referred to as the "gross misconduct" of an employee of the Library. Twelve months passed, and on January 25, 1939 a trustee committee reported a draft of rules "governing the conduct" of the Director which was returned to it for further study. On February 17 the full board requested Mr. Ballard's resignation in writing, "to be acted upon at such time as they see fit." President Davis reported on March 20 that he had it in hand. These remarkable actions were recorded without elaboration in the minutes, and nothing further was noted. One trustee recalls, however, that an employee was discovered taking his pleasure in the stacks. "There was considerable lively discussion in the Board because apparently Ballard was aware of this and had done nothing about it. It was the Board's opinion that this was improper conduct for an employee on company time."

Dr. Richard Goodwin Wadsworth, treasurer since 1918, died in 1936, closing a family era of sixty-one years of continuous service to the Boston Medical Library which began with his father, Dr. Oliver Fairfield Wadsworth, the founding secretary in 1875, and continued upon his resignation in 1911 with his son's election to the committee on library and finance. Members of the Wadsworth family contributed $10,000 to complete the executive offices in memory of father and son. Dr. Wadsworth was succeeded as treasurer by Dr. William C. Quinby.

Dr. Farlow died on September 24, 1937. He was eighty-four. President Davis said of him that "it was owing largely to his enthusiastic devotion and wise management that this collection of medical literature was built up from a small but valuable one to one of the outstanding medical libraries in the country."[18] Wrote a peer in the Medical Library Association: "Many of the members of this Association will remember his dignified manner, his graciousness and the pleasant twinkle in his eye when a bit of dry humor escaped his lips. There was some of the stern Puritan in his make-up, softened by an active interest in literature, art and especially music, for he was an accomplished pianist. . . His generous gifts to the Library for building and maintenance were much appreciated by a Board of Trustees who had more money for books than for equipment and cleaning."[19] Openhanded to the last, Dr. Farlow left his beloved BML $10,000 without restrictions.

Four months after the passing of the second librarian, the third, Dr. Charles F. Painter, retired after ten years of it. Henry R. Viets, a member of the library committee, was elected to succeed him at the annual meeting in January 1938. Dr. Viets's involvement with his mentor, Harvey Cushing, in the founding of the Boston Medical History Club has been mentioned, and it was as an avocational student of medical history, with a bachelor's leisure time from his neurological practice, that he assumed the librarianship.

Henry Viets was born in Lynn on March 7, 1890. He was graduated from Dartmouth College in 1912 and Harvard Medical School in 1916, then studied a year with Osler at Oxford as a Moseley Travelling Fellow. After army medical service he joined the Harvard faculty as a lecturer on neurology, and the neurology staff at the Massachusetts General Hospital with a special interest in myasthenia gravis. In 1935 he was the first at the MGH to use neostigmine in its treatment, and four years later he and his associates established the first myasthenia gravis clinic in the world there.

But the scholar in Viets was happiest. In 1930 he published *A Brief History of Medicine in Massachusetts*,[20] and since 1927 he had been on the editorial board of *The New England Journal of Medicine* and wrote regularly for it. Another medical historian who knew him well, Dr. Benjamin Spector, observed Osler's influence on Viets. . . that he "lived his life in the Oslerian spirit of litterae, scientia, praxis and doctrina"—and Cushing's. . . "crucial and indelible." From indifference to the serious study of medical history while a student, "the final transformation was brought about at the moment when Harvey Cushing opened, 'as gently as an obstetrician with a new-born babe,' a copy of the *Fabrica* of Vesalius which had been given to the Boston Medical Library by Osler. This unique experience, under the wing of a distinguished medical humanist-scholar, turned Henry Viets first into a neophyte, then an amateur, and finally into a professional in the history of medicine."[21]

The new Librarian's first annual report revealed that he held to rather more liberal views concerning the advantages of an affiliation with a certain unnamed medical school than any of his predecessors:[22]

> If it were not for the assistance afforded by the director, it would be impossible for an individual so poorly trained as myself to assume such an important office. The director's long acquaintance with the library and his expert knowledge of the technical details of running it removes from the librarian's shoulders nearly all of the load; the librarian need only supervise in general the library collection. His task, therefore, is quite different from that of most librarians, who serve as both librarian and director. This plan has, in the past, been in vogue in this library, and it is not at all uncertain that in the future a full-time position of librarian and possibly a teacher of medical history in a medical school might be advantageously combined. This, too, might lead more naturally to the bringing together of important collections of medical books in Boston. It is hoped that the future may bring such a plan into being, for the ultimate aim of the situation should be to create one center for all medical libraries, except those definitely associated with hospitals. This idea is not a new one. Enthusiasm for it, however, waxes and wanes from year to year. It must, I think, always be kept before us.

In reviving the subject of merger, Dr. Viets was not speaking on his own account alone. Lincoln Davis had already broken with the chauvinist tradition of past presidents by daring heresy in his 1935 report when he inveighed against the profession's lacklustre financial support, which he attributed partly to the Depression and in part to the growth of adequate working libraries in the medical schools and larger hospitals, and went on to conjecture:[23]

> It would seem that in a large medical centre such as Boston is, that a central medical library upon which smaller working libraries may draw is a most desirable economic arrangement. The question is can such an institution depend for adequate support on private endowment and membership. A library to progress with the times requires a very large endowment. Where is such an endowment coming from in these times? History seems to show that it is the libraries supported by National Governments or their sub-divisions, or large universities, which survive and progress. Has the time come when the Boston Medical Library should look to University affiliation to insure support and progress for the future?
>
> A central medical library affiliated with a great university and located within easy access to its medical students, with its facilities open to other schools as well, and to the medical profession at large, would seem an ideal which might appeal to some future benefactor.

This was 1935. That spring David Edsall retired as Dean of Harvard Medical School. In July 1936 his successor, Dr. C. Sidney Burwell, advised President Davis that a University committee had been appointed to consider closer affiliation between the School and the Boston Medical Library. That autumn the trustees of the BML received an informal legal opinion that affiliation with another institution was, after all, feasible.[24]

The first sign that the leaders of the two establishments had arrived secretly at some sort of open covenant appears in the form of a memorandum, appended to the trustees' minutes, of an informal meeting of physicians held at Dr. Davis's Beacon Street home on March 22, 1937. It was represented as a gathering of individuals concerned with the bibliothecarial interests of the amicable old adversaries. Present were Davis, Burwell, Painter, Viets, Fitz, George R. Minot, Francis M. Rackemann and Director Blake of the Harvard University Library. All but Blake were Fellows of the BML and graduates of Harvard Medical School, and every one but Painter was a present or former Harvard faculty member; it was agreed that he should represent the interests of the Tufts Medical School, and that Fitz should don a third hat and mind those of Boston University's, where he was also on the faculty. It was the plighting of a troth—some might have said a capitulation—which required but a dowry for its consummation. In the words of the memorandum:

> The general sense of this meeting was that it would be extremely desirable if

arrangements could be made at some future date to have in one building one medical library in Boston which would represent all the various medical library interests of the community. The first step in such a direction necessitates the Boston Medical Library and the Harvard Medical School Library acting from now on as one unit as far as is possible, for in all probability money will not be found in the immediate future to build a sufficiently large building for this general purpose. On the other hand, at least the idea should be kept in mind in the hope that when some donor or donors are found who are interested in a community enterprise of this general character, well-considered plans should be available for their consideration.

The gathering on Beacon Street agreed that, short of a new building, the two ought to endeavor to develop "to a certain extent as a joint library" with the first goal of avoiding unnecessary duplication. A committee representing the various medical libraries of Boston would be assembled to survey the shelves in the area and minimize duplication of acquisitions as a going policy toward the end that "the foundation for security in the future of one strong medical library would be established . . . and a considerable amount of money might well be saved by which to make the entire Boston medical library system stronger."

Dr. Davis and his guests of the evening pledged to seek the approval of the four institutions they represented in varying degrees. This was secured in principle from the BML trustees, who in October empowered their president to appoint a committee to meet with Harvard, and presumably from Harvard, Tufts and BU, because in the spring of 1938 Viets, Fitz and Castleman met with John Homans, chairman of the Harvard delegation (with Dean Burwell and Keyes Metcalf, the new Harvard College Librarian and Director of the University Library) and mapped out their first areas of agreement: the School would turn over all its dissertations to the Medical Library in return for the latter's public health reports.

Meanwhile, the WPA's Union Catalogue survey of the whereabouts of the area's medical literature had been approved and was under way. The joint library committee continued to meet at intervals. Early in 1939 the conferees agreed that the Medical Library would concentrate on clinical, historical and classical material, Harvard on biology and public health.[25] It was progress toward detente, and in his report to the annual meeting on January 28, 1941 at which he handed over the presidency to Dr. David Cheever, Lincoln Davis could applaud his library's cordial relations with the medical schools and larger hospitals and the reduction of competition and duplication in its relations with Harvard in particular. Cordial as they were, however, they presented "a difficult problem that awaits satisfactory solution. These smaller libraries provide for the ordinary needs of their clientele, so that many doctors do not feel the need of becoming members of the Boston Medical Library. What the ideal setup should be for this community needs serious study and wise decision. Preliminary steps in this study are already under way."[26]

Those first, faltering steps had first been assayed in 1936, when the Carnegie Corporation's possible interest in surveying the Boston medical library situation had been sounded out by Dr. Hans Zinsser; he drew a blank. Dr. Alan Gregg had then been approached at the Rockefeller Foundation, and indicated interest, but nothing came of it.[27] Three and a half years elapsed, when Harvard Librarian Keyes Metcalf, a member of the joint medical library committee, in January of 1940 asked the Carnegie Corporation for the humble sum of $1000 for the project. His request was approved in April, but it was not until 1941 that Thomas P. Fleming, Medical Librarian of the College of Physicians and Surgeons at Columbia University, was able to begin the study for which he had been commissioned.

As they had periodically during its history, it appeared that the planets were once again arranging themselves in a juxtaposition favorable to the destiny of the Boston Medical Library. Once again, however, clouds gathered upon the horizon.

10

Modernism's Grim Touch
1941 · 1955

This library is now faced with the serious problem of adjusting itself to new conditions. Should it remain the "gentleman's" library of the past, where tradition still is the important factor, or shoud it expand its services to meet the changing conditions which confront it? Upon this decision will rest the determination of the future of medical library facilities in Boston.

From the *Fleming Report*, 1941[1]

The Carnegie survey of medical libraries in Boston undertaken a few months before Pearl Harbor by Thomas P. Fleming, the Librarian of the College of Physicians and Surgeons at Columbia, was the first since that inventory of 1876 which convinced James Read Chadwick that the city needed one. Fleming's premise was that the old reliance on the academy or society library had been giving way since the mid-Twenties to the working institutional libraries whose growth was quickened by the expansion of research and the literature, the emphasis on reading in medical education and the rise of the medical centers with their need for ready reference. Utilization of central libraries, however, had generally not diminished in the face of this trend, but on the contrary—with the notable exception of Boston—had kept pace with it. In Fleming's view, medical schools and hospitals in large metropolitan areas ought to maintain working libraries only for their daily purposes so long as a large back-up reference collection was at hand.

The major hospital libraries of Boston were in the main serving well, Fleming found. Not so the medical schools. Least satisfactory was the Tufts Medical College library, where the clinical sciences especially were so poorly represented as to compromise the school's educational objectives, a deficiency he hoped would be corrected if and when Tufts moved into the New England Medical Center complex in the South End. The library of the Boston University School of Medicine he graded fair in the basic and good in the clinical sciences, but under pressure from the necessity of doubling for the staff of the adjacent Massachusetts Memorial Hospitals. The central library of the Harvard Medical School had benefitted from the cooperative efforts with the Boston Medical Library, but it was short on stack and reading space, and seriously short on staff; Fleming urged the integration of the remaining departmental libraries in physiology-biochemistry, anatomy and legal medicine. Relatively close as they were to 8 The Fenway, the schools and hospitals comprising what he called the Harvard Medical Center were yet too distant for the BML to furnish the immediate needs of house staff, particularly; hence Harvard had been forced to develop independently.

Fleming expectedly praised the collections of the Medical Library, and regretted the aching void of stackless space in the unfinished addition. His reference to the "gentlemen's club" and his observations about its atmosphere and staff, not surprisingly, were *not* singled out for inclusion in the Library's next annual report. To the surveyor,

> the appearance of antiquity which unfortunately permeates the building unconsciously suggests a drab, somewhat unfriendly and forbidding atmosphere. . . The staff consists of the Director, a Secretary, the Librarian and three assistants (reference, circulation and cataloguing) and two boys on duty at night. The position of Librarian is an administrative one. He serves without pay and his work does not entail any active participation in the technical processes or services to readers. The reference and circulation assistants "page" all the books and shelve most of them. The cataloguer makes no use of the facilities of the Library of Congress for printed cards. She assigns subject headings under the direction of the Director who personally classifies all books. In order to render more effective service, the staff needs to be considerably enlarged. Clerks should be provided to handle the routine work so that experienced assistants would be free to perform the function for which they were employed. Steps should be taken at once to prevent the inevitable chaotic conditions which would result if the present Director should become incapacitated. An assistant to the Director should be appointed in order to absorb the tremendous knowledge which he possesses. The staff has been so inadequate that much which in other libraries is a matter of documentary record is carried solely in the Director's head.[2]

The Columbia librarian did not reserve his criticism for the largest and the leading. The administration, and utilization, of every medical library in Boston were below the national mean, he discovered, reflecting their failure to furnish adequate reading, bibliographic and reference facilities, access to their collections and instruction in their use, sufficient copies of literature in heavy demand, and messenger service to laboratories.[3] As to why, Fleming did not offer an opinion. He did not mention the effect of the Depression on budgets and staffs, which was, of course, national. Boston stodginess, perhaps.

> There is no doubt that the newer libraries are meeting the immediate demands of a major portion of the medical profession, and, as a consequence, it has been assumed that this explains why the use of the Boston Medical Library has not greatly increased while that of the other medical libraries has shown constant

growth. Further it seems natural to assume that physicians may question themselves as to the advantages to be gained by taking out or continuing membership in the Boston Medical Library when their individual demands for medical literature are being adequately supplied by the medical school or hospital libraries. If these assumptions are true, then support for the Boston Medical Library will continue to fall off, and this splendid collection, which is unexcelled in many fields and vitally essential for the practising physician and research worker alike, will face a somewhat uncertain future.[4]

The other two members of the survey committee to which Fleming reported his findings—Dr. John F. Fulton, Sterling Professor of Physiology at Yale, and Dr. Nye, editor of *The New England Journal of Medicine*—joined in recommending that the Boston Medical Library in future confine its function to that of a regional reference facility, that its staff be increased, and that a substantial fund be raised either to erect a new building altogether for a "New England Academy of Medicine" to house the BML, the Massachusetts Medical Society and the *Journal*, or, alternatively, to modernize 8 The Fenway, finish off the stack addition and fatten the endowment.

Having raised the questions, Lincoln Davis left the answers to his successors and relinquished the presidency to David Cheever at the annual meeting in January 1941. Cheever was the brilliant son of an illustrious father, David Williams Cheever, president from 1896 to 1906. Born in 1876, he was graduated from Harvard College with high honors and from its Medical School, where his father was a professor of surgery, in 1901. By way of the teaching of anatomy, then general surgery, and its practise, he followed the track of his sire. The son was on the organizing staff of the Brigham with Cushing, the visiting staff at City Hospital, and in time Professor of Surgery at Harvard himself, only to be brought down in his prime by severe arthritis. Cheever resigned the chair of surgery in 1939; the next year he was elected a Harvard overseer, and then to the head of the Library. "His brave attitude toward his crippling and painful disease attests to his moral and physical courage," wrote an associate. "His home life was ideal for a man who enjoyed children and grandchildren, saddened only by the death of his devoted wife about the time of his retirement. As a social being he was an ideal companion at work or play, and his intimates claim that they never heard him utter an unkind word about others."[5]

America was in World War II when Dr. Cheever reviewed the situation of the Medical Library at the annual meeting in March 1942. The Fleming Report had shaken up the trustees. They regarded the future of the Library (as not a few did the world's) with *grave anxiety*. "The Library looks well-nourished and presents—with some reservations—

an outward appearance of health, but its intimate advisers know that it is anaemic and that its vital organs are suffering from financial anoxemia." There were the very largely unfinished stacks, the hopeless backlog of material, the bare-bone budget, the skeleton staff, and yes, out with it. . . "our Director, completing his 50th year of continuous service, must be supposed to be mortal—ageless though he seems—and his accumulated experience and knowledge should be communicated to a young associate."

In wartime more than ever, Cheever reminded the Fellows, planning for the future must not go by the board.

> As a Nation we are literally in a death-grapple with an implacable, relentless and powerful foe whose purpose is to enslave us, and it is quite likely many of us may say that this is no time to bother about matters which seem to have no relation to the struggle we are making to win the war, but surely on further thought every man of us will realize that this is the time of all others when we must guard and hold fast that which is good, and which has been amply proved to be a source of strength and inspiration.[6]

The second World War in a generation jolted America out of its Depression. In the early stages there was genuine concern that the Germans might attack the eastern seaboard, and the more valuable possessions of the Boston Medical Library were moved to shelter. For the second time in twenty-five years the Teutonic tourniquet was twisted around the flow of foreign scientific periodicals. Only the British and Russian journals trickled through.[7] An exchange with twenty-seven from the Soviet Union was kept up throughout the war; these were supplemented by Harvard's, and it was agreed that the BML should be the repository of Slavic medical literature in Boston.

When the Oil Rationing Board announced in December 1942 that it could assure only fuel enough to keep the Library open one week a month, the Boston Edison Company piped in spent steam from its generators, a reprieve which increased operating costs and lost the BML the $1100 the Massachusetts Historical Society had been paying annually for its own surplus. But President Cheever was thankful for small blessings. "We are grateful that we are warmed and sheltered, and able to pursue our work with no more serious interruptions than practice air-raid alarms."[8]

Attendance in 1943 was down a third from 1942, largely due to the claims of the services on 159 members. They took their dues with them by vote of the trustees, a patriotic remittance which meant deficits for the duration and longer when combined with raises for the staff and the failure of investment income to recover its old levels. Mrs. Annie

Farlow died in 1943, matching her late husband's bequest of $10,000, unrestricted and as welcome in this conflict as the elevator she had provided for the "less active and more short-winded" of the older members at the end of the last one.

Hours previously the infantry and tanks of the British Eighth Army had jumped off on the great drive toward El Alamain, when on October 24, 1942 James Francis Ballard observed the fiftieth anniversary of his employment as Dr. Brigham's errand boy. The Boston Medical Library put on a reception for its Director, his *semi-centennial*, as President Cheever was pleased to describe an occasion honoring an institution within an institution. Nevertheless, he was careful not to over-flatter one who at sixty-four persisted in the methodical cultivation of his indispensability. Mr. Ballard has served continuously and efficiently, observed the President, "educating himself in the technique of library administration, acquiring a familiarity with medical literature and a knowledge of medical bibliophilism, that has placed him in the front rank of medical librarians in this country and won him the position of Director of the Library."[9] Still that trace of condescension. Back in 1914, in his first publication, "Some Problems in the Administration of a Medical Library," the object of the day's congratulations had turned the needle on his patrons: "The power of selection and purchasing should be vested in the librarian [and he did *not* mean Dr. Farlow] . . .The average physician is the last person to whom the task of selecting books should be entrusted."[10]

A colleague in the Medical Library Association in which (Jim to some, James to others) Ballard had served in most official and many unofficial capacities, W. B. McDaniel 2d, Librarian of the College of Physicians of Philadelphia, sized him up as a "shrewd, occasionally exasperating, but fundamentally warm-hearted pioneer," indeed the dean of the profession and the prototype for the classic description of the species once promulgated by the Association's Bulletin: "The medical librarian must have the agility of the robin, the eye of a hawk and the voice of a dove. When he refuseth it seemeth like conferring a favor. He loveth his books. He handleth a rare old volume like a newborn babe. The waste of time is unknown to him. He knoweth that while he listeneth to a tedious recital he can figure where the money is coming from to mend that leak in the roof." To these ornithoid characteristics might be added a measure of owlishness perceived (though not explicitly) by McDaniel: "Serene in manner (he claimed that he never took the day's troubles home with him), with arms usually crossed while he was standing, head tilted a little back, Mr. Ballard talked and listened attentively, with little facial expression to vary the faintly sardonic natural one—yet apparently missed little, of flora or fauna, visible around him."[11]

Long before his *semi-centennial* the Director's personality had so interlaced itself with that of his Library that each was regarded by Ballard-watchers as the alter ego of the other. He had the politician's facility for getting along with whomever he needed to, and the frankness to admit that he had an equal facility for masking his private opinions. At the meetings of the Medical Library Association, as McDaniel remarked, "if a sound step forward was proposed, a quiet word from him, uttered at a strategically favorable moment, might well decide .the question. Not above an occasional non sequitur himself, he benignly tolerated those of the rest of us, unless one of his sleepless antennae warned him that one of his objectives might be endangered. A parliamentarian by nature, he could either disrupt a meeting by abruptly phrased objections to the procedure; or, if friendship or other factors so counseled remain silent and at a later date see that justice was done to his principles." His larger interests notwithstanding, "it may be that Mr. Ballard had only one deep and unquestioning loyalty, that to his library—which might, in a sense, be regarded as an extension of himself. He could be kind and affectionate in his reserved way over long periods of time, as many of us will long and gratefully remember. But all other professional attachments than the one, it seems possible, were monitored in its interest."[12]

Anticipating the golden moment of their Director, the trustees established the James F. Ballard Publication Fund "to make better known to its friends the treasures and resources of the Library." The initial productions were appropriately his, both appearing in 1944. The first was the summation of the closest of the close to his heart, a compilation of the collection of incunabula which had now reached 674, together with fifty-two rare manuscripts, entitled *A Catalogue of the Medieval and Renaissance Manuscripts and Incunabula in the Boston Medical Library*, with a scholarly introduction and appraisal by Dr. Viets, assigning 541 of the incunables to the Bullard Collection, thirty-one to the Hyams Fund, five to the John Warren Fund and ninety-seven to the general funds of the Library. The collection as a whole was believed to fulfill Dr. Bullard's aim of duplicating the library of a learned physician of the late fifteenth century in Europe. The assistance of Dr. Arnold C. Klebs, the eminent medical incunabulist, was acknowledged. Bibliographically, the major credit for this achievement belonged to Ballard, especially in the years since Bullard's death. But the erudite and often amusing commentaries in the *Catalogue*, presented in the zestful vein which made treatises of his annual reports, were the work of Henry Viets.

James Ballard was a fair appraiser, of books, men and self. He addressed a meeting of the Boston chapter of the Special Libraries Association in 1936 thus: "My personal interests are general biography, medieval history and customs, bibliography in general and in particular of incunabula and books printed in 17th and 16th centuries, library administration and library technique in all of its branches. . . I am known as an authority on the value of early printed medical books, and the classics of medicine, and I am consulted by book-dealers, librarians and individuals and I am glad to be of help in such matters."[13] This fleeting revelation of self-image interested the observant Philadelphia librarian:

> In the light of Mr. Ballard's keen sense of temporal values, it might be thought that this expressed interest, frequently demonstrated, in the historical area of medicine, was a dutifully cultivated one. This would possibly be, in part, true. The man who "handleth a rare old volume like a newborn babe" might, conceivably, have no more elevating thought in mind than the cost of replacing it. But those who knew Mr. Ballard will probably agree that his interest went deeper than the call of duty required. The interest in rare books, in medieval history and customs, represented, let us say, a sincerely felt avocation that had the good fortune to serve well the vocation. . . His famous "Catalogue of the Medieval and Renaissance Manuscripts and Incunabula in the Boston Medical Library" (1944) is perhaps the most eloquent demonstration of, simultaneously, the Director's superb talents as a collector of historical documents and of his quite accountable weaknesses in describing their contents in terms unexceptionable to those most likely to make use of them. It was not, one willingly believes, a case of the Wilde-ian fellow who knew the price of everything and the value of nothing; but, rather, an instance of our human and very common failure sometimes to assess ruthlessly the limits of our own competence.[14]

Still, rather well done for a chap whose formal education ceased during the first weeks of the eighth grade. In searching for the source of Ballard's medievalism, incidentally, one need hardly look beyond that cavalier knight-errant of his youth, Jim Chadwick.

The second of the publications generated by the Director's fifty years of service was the third edition of *The Boston Medical Library Medical Classification*, whose 1925 edition of 772 copies had long been exhausted. Part I, *Schedules*, appeared in 1944, followed by the *Index*, Part II, in 1946. The twenty years of scientific advance and additions to the literature which separated the printings had modified the author's enthusiasm for the shelf divisions of simpler days. "Classification is limited means toward the objective of thoroughly organized literature. It never can take the place of extensive subject and author cataloguing and is useful only for open-access collections. Classification is the least important of major library processes. . . A fetish should not be made of classification and its expansion carried to the extreme where a separate niche is provided for practically every single book or pamphlet in the collection."[15]

The dangerous dependence of the Boston Medical Library on the well-being of its aging Director ("though he has done better," President Cheever hastened to protest, "than Ponce de Leon in his search for the mythical fountain"[16]) had been warned against in the Fleming Report, but although the annual budgets produced deficits, they contained no Keynesian solutions to the affliction of underemployment in the line of succession.

The academy of medicine route to the future proposed as one alternative in the Fleming Report was again scouted in the spring of 1942 by the interested parties, including "Boston medicine in general" represented by Dr. Roger I. Lee. Even the Overseers' Committee to visit the Harvard Medical School, of which David Cheever was chairman, got involved with a discussion of the notion that the BML might glamorize itself with prospective members and donors by changing its name to the "Boston Academy of Medicine."[17] The path was swallowed in a jungle of obstacles, however. Perhaps the decisive demurrer was thrown across it by Keyes Metcalf, the Harvard Librarian, who, after inspecting the premises on The Fenway, threw his weight to the conservative alternative proposed by the Fleming committee. He expressed some surprise at the relative adequacy of the structure and thought it would do for another twenty-five or thirty years if $100,000 could be raised to install the stacks, and another $10,000 in annual income, mainly for an expanded staff. An academy of medicine he considered financially out of the question.[18]

Dr. Cheever reviewed the war-weary year of 1944 with discouragement. The deficit for the twelve months was over $3000. Any hope for financial help from an agency or foundation would depend upon the matching generosity of the members and the community, and the Library was stagnating. "Unlike the orchid, it cannot live on air and admiration; the founders rooted it sturdily in the soil, and on the soil it must continue to depend for its support."[19]

Toward the end of 1944 Metcalf offered to approach the Rockefeller Foundation for a capital grant of $50,000 on a matching basis which he proposed should be contingent on an annual subsidy of roughly $10,000 from the three Boston medical schools and possibly the larger hospitals, and most important (as he stressed to Cheever and Viets), on the hiring of an assistant to understudy Ballard. In the spring of 1945 the trustees approved what was now being called the Fleming-Metcalf Plan. But in the autumn Metcalf reported that he had been given no encouragement by the Rockefeller Foundation and other sources he had sounded out and declared his belief that the plan could not be funded. Discouraged himself now, he suggested the Library retrench by restricting its reserve collections. The board concluded it had no course but to reject again the academy proposition and to table indefinitely, at best, the alternative put forward by the Fleming committee and enlarged upon by Metcalf.[20]

One remaining source of operating income, the organized medical profession of Massachusetts, had not been tapped. For years an alliance with the Massachusetts Medical Society had been the object of desultory suit. Suddenly, as dreams of wealthy angels faded, the courtship was resumed with unwonted ardor on the initiative of Dr. Walter G. Phippen of Salem, a newcomer to the trustees. Presuming that the BML ought to increase its annual income from $32,000 to at least $60,000 before committing itself to a new program, he proposed to the board in April 1945 that an effort be made to persuade the 5000 Fellows of the Society to assess themselves five dollars a year for the Library's sake, just as they had come to the rescue when the *Journal* was in financial trouble.[21]

Phippen was in a strategic position to make the overture. He had been the Society's president from 1939 to 1941, then president of the New England Surgical Society, and enjoyed the unusually warm respect and affection of his colleagues, to whom at sixty-eight he was an elder statesman of uncommon judgment. His living monument was the Salem Hospital where he had started in general practise in 1907 by way of Harvard College and Medical School, the MGH and a year in Vienna. After its devastation in the great Salem fire of 1914, Dr. Phippen took the lead in its rebuilding in 1917 and in making of it a national model of the modern community hospital.

As World War II ended, and the world aligned anew, the matter of some formal understanding between the Boston Medical Library and the Massachusetts Medical Society came under renewed discussion. At the annual meeting on March 5, 1946 David Cheever passed along the holding operation over which he had presided for five years to his logical successor, Walter Phippen, with the first hopefulness he had been able to muster:

> The broad and liberal view seems to be that we have two organizations whose purposes are essentially identical in striving to promote the public health, each with an enviable record of unselfish service over many years. The one has a plant and collections of stored medical knowledge second to but few in this country but lacks endowment and other income adequate for its support; the other through its numerical strength and wide influence is able to contribute that

support. As one who for nearly 45 years has been active in the affairs of both these organizations and who has the deep conviction that the prestige and strength of each would be promoted by a close alliance, I have no hesitation in urging that its feasibility be explored to the end that its consummation be accomplished at the earliest possible moment, for time is of the essence now that after the disruption of the World War the institutes of peace are to be restored.[22]

President Phippen broached the delicate subject of subsidy with the executive committee of the Medical Society so convincingly that on February 7, 1947 the Council raised the dues from twenty to twenty-five dollars, on the condition that for their extra five some form of membership in the Library be conferred upon the Fellows. It was done; a special meeting of the Boston Medical Library on November 17 amended the by-laws to create a new class of "Massachusetts Medical Society Members"—namely, any resident Fellow of the Society, active or retired, in good standing on January 1, 1948—adding four Society-appointed trustees to the existing board of twelve, and establishing the office of assistant treasurer.

By this late-blooming marriage the Library overnight increased its operating income by seventy per cent and its membership by nearly fivefold, and put itself in a fair way to embarking on the crash diet and fitness regimen which Keyes Metcalf had laid down for it in anticipation of the joyous, if autogamous, union (almost to a person, the Fellows of the Library were Fellows of the Society).

First of all, Metcalf advised, the old accessions policy of trying to maintain a universal collection should be abandoned for the narrower objective of reference only. Unwanted nonmedical books and journals should be discarded, and outmoded texts and back files of periodicals should be moved into storage which was now available in the New England Deposit Library that Harvard had built on Western Avenue behind its Business School. These two measures, Metcalf believed, would shake down the Library for many more years of service on the Fens. He outlined six additional steps: put the rest of the collection in order; refurnish and improve the lighting in Holmes Hall; cull and catalogue the mess in the basement and its ubiquitous overflow; complete the Union Catalogue; consider remaining open evenings and Sundays; set up a pension plan for the older employees and recruit a vigorous young staff to reorganize the Library.[23]

In January 1947 the trustees approved the first two steps of the new Metcalf Plan after being advised by Dr. Viets that a quarter of one floor at the Deposit Library—room for 20,000 volumes, about ten per cent of the shelf at the BML—would be available after July 1 at a yearly rent of

$1150; as many again could be thrown out. In his annual report that March the Librarian roughed out his revised accessional objectives: files of around a thousand current medical periodicals, the latest texts and monographs, and current editions of well-accepted publications, emphasis on clinical medicine; current works in allied fields, supplemented by interlibrary loans; and a practical sampling of the great works in the history of medicine. . . "this, however, would not be the primary interest of the Library and the Librarian does not contemplate turning the Boston Medical Library into an antiquarian society." Viets welcomed the just-pledged financial bonanza from the Massachusetts Medical Society:

> The Library is primarily an educational institution, devoted to the education of the doctor of our time. Every book and pamphlet on our shelves is of interest to someone, but the greatest use of the Library naturally comes with the current literature of all lands and in this we are, indeed, fortunate in the large number of journals, transactions of societies, and reports which we accumulate year by year. With the cooperation of the other libraries in and near Boston the Library expects in the near future to be able to make available for the laboratory worker, specialist and the general practitioner all the current literature that is worthwhile. Every book and journal may not find a place on the shelves of the Boston Medical Library, but should that work be available in Boston or, indeed, anywhere in the United States, the Boston Medical Library will bring it to the doctor's desk or his laboratory table.[24]

Dr. Robert N. Nye, the editor of *The New England Journal of Medicine* who had succeeded Dr. William C. Quinby as treasurer in 1946, died on September 10, 1947 and was replaced by the cardiologist Howard B. Sprague, a trustee. Dr. Joseph Garland, an associate editor for twenty-five years, retired from the practise of pediatrics and a brief secretaryship of the Medical Socety to edit the *Journal*; a trustee since March, he was appointed the Library's first assistant treasurer in January 1948.

Braced by the urgings of Fleming and Metcalf, the board resolved in the fall of 1947 to consider retiring Director Ballard, now fifty-five years with the BML and pushing seventy, and finding a successor. Probably in reaction, he enlarged his staff by two and declared his intention of hiring two more when he could find qualified candidates. The following February the trustees discussed possibilities for his replacement, inconclusively. That October they offered the position of assistant to the Director and reference librarian (succeeding Miss Catherine L. Binderup)[25] to Charles C. Colby III, explicitly without assurance that he was heir apparent. Colby was twenty-five, a native of Newark, New Jersey, and a graduate of Harvard College, and of Simmons College in library science. He had finished his first year at Harvard Medical School after entering military service, from which he was discharged in 1946. Since July 1947 he had been a subject cataloguer at the Army Medical Library. In November he accepted the offer of the trustees and came to work at 8 The Fenway in January 1949.

While the officers of the Boston Medical Library puffed valiantly at the dust of three quarters of a century, their tenants, who were suffused with the postwar surge of new blood and energy, grew restless. For a while the Medical Society considered reconstructing the offices on the first floor. In the spring of 1949 Bradford Washburn created some stir when he invited Library and Society to relocate next to his new Boston Museum of Science on the Charles River Dam; the Library was mildly interested, and it stopped at that.[26] In 1950 the Society purchased the former Peabody town house at 22 The Fenway and moved in the next year after extensive renovation which turned the ground floor of the stack addition of the Library over to its *Journal*, and the former administrative offices of the Society to *The Journal of Bone and Joint Surgery* and the Medical Advisory Board of the Selective Service Advisory Committee for Massachusetts.

The liaison with the Medical Society was having some effects which were not entirely anticipated. The income from the increased dues of the doctors of the Commonwealth in 1950, the Library's seventy-fifth anniversary, was $27,395, or thirty-seven per cent of a budget which finished $5125 in the black. This blessing was faintly mixed with a decline of $1550 in regular dues since 1947 as the result of a net loss of sixty-six members, most of whom felt there was nothing to be gained by voluntarily paying twenty dollars for what they got for their compulsory five. President Phippen was not unsympathetic: "From a strictly practical point of view we must be fair and say that the fellowship does not bring fifteen dollars' worth of extra service. We wish that some way might be found for library fellowship to carry special privileges. Many schemes have been suggested, such as a sort of literary club with special rooms set apart—an Academy of Medicine and so forth—but none of them have materialized." He appealed to the highmindedness of the profession. By 1951, when the roster had shrunk by another seventy-eight, he thought the frugality of his brethren "incredible."[27]

While members were grappling with their consciences over the dues option, they were getting their money's worth in spades from the Librarian's offer of 1947 to bring any medical work in existence to their desks. Attendance had increased predictably from 9158 in 1947 to 13,775 in 1950; but during the same period circulation and use of the collections had escalated beyond all expectations from 42,638 to 64,256, the major part of which was attributed to the Medical Society members, a lesser portion to the professional category which had increased from thirty-two in 1946 to forty-one in 1950, including twenty-six hospitals and clinics, the three medical schools, various libraries and government agencies, and three businesses.

The manner of the admission to membership of one of the latter, the since-defunct Lydia E. Pinkham Medicine Company of Lynn, is strangely obscure. The firm's application had been rejected by the trustees on April 15, 1940 on the ground that Mrs. Pinkham's vegetable compound for female ailments was listed in neither the *United States Pharmacopeia* nor *New and Nonofficial Remedies* of the American Medical Association. Three years passed, when most unobtrusively and without a word of mention in the board minutes the nostrum manufacturer turned up on the list of professional members in the 1943 annual report and from that year on for as long as they were printed. The Library's records are mute. The fact is that in 1938 the Food and Drug Administration had relayed to the Federal Trade Commission (which was interesting itself in such matters) the opinion that the Pinkham compound was at most a mild stomachic tonic. The FTC opened negotiations with the maker, as with other patent medicine manufacturers, and after more than two years agreed in January 1941 that it could continue advertising so long as it abandoned its former claims that the product had any more than a symptomatic effect on female functional disorders. This grudging approval by a Federal agency may have been the ticket that admitted Mrs. Pinkham so covertly through the rear door of 8 The Fenway.[28]

The strain on the staff of the kind of service which made professional membership so desirable caused the Librarian to admit that the complications of the alliance with the Medical Society were beyond anything imagined and had brought on numerous problems which were beginning to outweigh the financial dividends.[29] Viets wanted to give more time to the Library himself, and to get paid for it.

The diamond jubilee had featured historical exhibits in the rotunda of 8 The Fenway and at the Boston Public Library, prepared by the Director, and a banquet at the Hotel Kenmore on October 18, 1950 at which the main speaker was Chauncey D. Leake, Dean of the Medical Program at the University of Texas. Henry Viets was the toastmaster, and it may have been with the hope of the good fellowship of the evening lasting through to the next trustees' meeting that he reminded them in a memorandum that on April 1, 1951 he would be sixty-one and retiring from the MGH and Harvard; he wanted to devote most of his energy to the Library, but to do so (since the position of Librarian traditionally was honorary but without honorarium) he would need $6000 a year for himself and a secretary. He retired, without a decision, and after waiting a seemly while raised the subject with Dr. Richard Warren, grandson of J. Collins Warren, who was carrying on the family tradition and had succeeded Benjamin Castleman as secretary in 1950. In October of 1951, at Warren's urging, the board picked Dr. Viets's request off the table and then laid it down again indefinitely, citing the Library's "precarious financial condition."[30]

The Medical Library's anniversary year of 1950 was also the anniversary, President Phippen informed the annual meeting in some exasperation, of the incompletion of the stack addition, its twentieth. Rental at the New England Deposit Library was now costing $2000 a year, the income from a principal of about $50,000. Now if someone would step forward with $50,000, three tiers of stack could be built, the Deposit Library could be vacated, and $2000 a year saved. "I do not know how many fellows of the Library appreciate the necessity of more stack room. At the risk of tiresome repetition let me say that the stack building was built in 1930 of substantial construction to contain seven sets of stacks. . . Two stacks only were constructed. . . An open elevator well was constructed, but no elevator installed. The two completed tiers were soon filled, and temporary scaffolding was erected, on which boxes upon boxes of books have been stacked upward and upward; to reach them requires the agility and sure-footedness of a Rocky Mountain goat. It can be readily understood without the necessity of seeing this wilderness that the arrangement does not work for efficiency. Furthermore, it is very wasteful of space."[31]

One who heeded the presidential voice crying from the wilderness, and thought he saw the promised land beyond somewhere, was Dr. Arthur W. Allen, the departing president of the Massachusetts Medical Society who had come on the board of trustees in 1949 after retiring from a lectureship in surgery at Harvard and twelve years as chief of the East Surgical Service at the MGH. Something had to be done, certainly. The Library had nowhere to retreat; it could not hold on to the status quo much longer; and without a very large infusion of money it could not go forward. The trustees were simply up against it. . . "aware," as Phippen conceded, "of our inability to properly evaluate the problem ourselves."[32]

Late in 1951 Arthur Allen suggested that expert advice be sought concerning the BML's fundraising capacity and the outlook for improved public relations (a term for the postwar institutional self-consciousness that was coming into vogue), upon which Dr. Phippen promptly appointed him chairman of an ad hoc reconstruction and financing committee with fellow trustees Robert W. Buck and John W. Norcross. These engaged Herbert L. Beckwith of the architectural firm of Anderson and Beckwith, which had supervised the renovation of the Medical Society's quarters, to examine the problems and potential of the Library, and they raised an "exploration fund" of $4327 among the Fellows to pay for the survey.

The Beckwith Report was submitted on May 7, 1952, and it was reassuring.[33] The surveyors found that most of the BML's patrons considered it indispensable to them. Comparison with three other regional medical libraries yielded the surprising information that its circulation was rising faster than that of the College of Physicians of Philadelphia, while the New York Academy of Medicine's and the Kings County Medical Society's in Brooklyn were actually falling. Attendance, also, at the BML had increased steadily since 1947 in the face of a decline at the other three. Analysis of these trends and of the opinions of the librarians of institutional members indicated that the BML could profit by broadening its base of participation, and hence of financial support, into the fields allied to medicine which were responsible for a large component of its expanding circulation. Moving a step beyond Fleming and Metcalf, Anderson and Beckwith recommended that the Library aim at developing as the New England research reference center in medicine and the rapidly expanding allied sciences, with renewed emphasis on accessions in the basic disciplines.

Even as Boston's use curve was climbing while New York's, Brooklyn's and Philadelphia's descended, so was the work load of the staff, whose ratio to patrons was found to be the lowest of the four. The librarians of the member institutions were unreserved in their praise of the overtaxed cadre, which they dissociated from its working conditions. As an example, the librarian at Boston University School of Medicine had seen titles not yet processed at the BML which were already dog-eared on her shelves. Their comments on 8 The Fenway "usually began with the use of one or more of the words 'dark,' 'gloomy,' 'depressing,' 'uncomfortable,' 'musty,' 'dusty,' 'crowded' or 'somber' before any specifics were mentioned."

Griminess was tops among the peeves of the librarians; they complained in particular about the "excessively heavy dirt cover on books retrieved from the bowels of the place. The frustration of trying to find parking space was unforgettable: the librarian of the Veterans Administration Hospital in West Roxbury limited requests there at any one time to six books, an armful, the most she or her driver could or would handle while double-parked outside. Three of the librarians admitted that they rather liked the somber and musty atmosphere of the BML; to a fourth, however, it was "not a place that calls to you;" to a scornful fifth it was "ancient but not honorable." And one young lady sent from the Massachusetts Eye and Ear Infirmary was "so frightened at BML entrance she fled."

Nevertheless, the consultants were optimistic that the most frequent criticisms of 8 The Fenway ("doesn't even have an authentic Boston flavor") regarding environment, layout and lighting could be met with four improvements:

1. Completion of the stacks	$210,203
2. Replacement of stairs and elevator to comply with building ordinance	200,673
3. Remodelling first and second floors	114,140
4. Remodelling John Ware Hall, adding a second exit required by law	70,028
Miscellaneous work	16,500
	$611,544

To Walter Phippen, who had already decided a bit sorrowfully, as he said, that six years in the presidency was enough, the Beckwith Report was "astounding." He was agreeably surprised upon learning of "the universal opinion among the users of the Library that its loss would greatly handicap all progress in medicine in this area for decades to come."[34] He then stepped down for Arthur Allen at the annual meeting on May 19, 1952 which had been moved from March to coincide with the Medical Society's.

"Jimmy" Allen was a softly drawlish Kentuckian out of Georgetown College and Johns Hopkins Medical School in 1913, sixty-four, four years retired, a former president of the American College of Surgeons (and of the Mass Medical Society), internationally honored, immensely popular. . . in short, the right man at the right time to coax, if anyone could, the Boston Medical Library in his urbane and persuasive way into the pastures of wider recognition, and then appreciation, which it was hoped would produce a harvest of green. Some ground had been turned over in a preliminary fashion during a series of teas put on in March to spread the gospel among presumably interested physicians and laymen by the device of safaris into the stackless wilderness so that they might see for themselves the enormity of the void. Soon after taking office Dr. Allen appointed an executive committee of the trustees consisting of himself, vice president, librarian, treasurer, secretary and Emeritus Phippen, to meet at frequent intervals in preparation for a possible campaign. During the summer this committee invited the New York fundraising firm of Marts and Lundy to conduct an exploratory survey.

The findings of the New Yorkers were laid before the trustees on December 12, 1952 and made it all too clear that neither virtue nor excellence nor a combination of the two was necessarily its own reward.[35] By the embarrassingly simple expedient of thumbing through the accounts, the firm revealed that in the fifteen years since 1937 the Library had received fifty-three gifts amounting to $9475 and six bequests of $13,967. During 1951 the sum total of twenty dollars had been contributed toward operating expenses. This dolorous record led the fundraisers to the gently-phrased conclusion that "obviously the friends of the Boston Medical Library do not have the Library in mind as they make their contributions to the philanthropic institutions which they support year by year. . . No administrative provision seems to exist for seeking financial support for the operation of the Library."

A sampling of physicians elicited a favorable attitude toward the BML and its needs, and an awareness of the profession's obligation to bear the brunt of its financial support. But of course that had proved long since insufficient. "In spite of the generations of useful and honorable service which the Boston Medical Library has rendered the community, it seems to have hidden its light under a bushel, and, consequently, the leaders of Boston community life, who are so sympathetic and generous toward many other forces for community betterment, feel no present sense of responsibility for the Boston Medical Library. . . It will be necessary to create out of whole cloth a giving constituency which does not now exist."

The firm recommended a low-pressure effort for six months to raise between $100,000 and $300,000 and to begin the cultivation of a wider group of supporters in the community from which to raise the balance of the larger objective over a period of years. Its fee for the short-term project would be $27,300.

On December 17, 1952 the trustees engaged Marts and Lundy to manage "The Boston Medical Library Greater Service Program." Initially the goal was set at one million dollars, including $510,000 for endowment. Early in 1953, when a fundraising brochure was in the making, the sights were raised to $1,250,000, to be sought in two stages: (1) a six-month target of $250,000 to fill the void with stacks, install an elevator, put in a file room, finish the periodical room and break through another fire exit from John Ware Hall, and (2) a long-range objective of another million dollars consisting of endowment of $750,000 for a larger staff and increased salaries, and $250,000 for remodeling the main entrance (in memory of that frightened, fleeing female from the Eye and Ear) and replacing Mrs. Farlow's elevator, the stairs, the plumbing and the wiring at Number 8.

Several hundred members and lay friends beat the brush under the professional direction of James H. Duchine and John I. Carlson in a well organized campaign, and it succeeded. By September of 1953 about $224,000 pledged by 967 contributors had financed completion of the alterations to Ware Hall. In December pledges reached $276,142, and the fundraisers departed. Work in the stack building was started. Dr. Charles H. Bradford, like his father, Edward, an orthopedist and devotee of the Library, in May 1954 headed a special development committee of those who had been active in the fund drive and wanted to see it through in the long pull. Before the end of June $306,000 had been pledged. That autumn, twenty-three years after work on the shell to surround them was abandoned, the six floors of new stacks were in place, the block and tackle had given way to an elevator, and the mighty job of disinterring, sorting out and moving in the miser's hoard had begun—a two-year project in the estimate of Director Ballard, who was entering briskly upon his sixty-third year on the job, quite unperturbed by the appointment a few months earlier of still another committee assigned to look for his successor.

Perhaps after all, in that interesting estimation of W. B. McDaniel, it was Mr. Ballard's "deep-rooted library-self identification, supported by a physical and mental vigor little affected by the years, that made it possible for him to, by his own characteristically frank account, make ineffective in late years the normal steps taken by an institution to avoid a potential administrative hiatus caused by the sudden incapacity of an important elderly executive. In this instance only may Mr. Ballard's supreme devotion to the interests of his library be thought to have faltered."[36]

Time intervened on his side. On Saturday the fourteenth of May, 1955, the Director spent the morning as usual at The Fenway, returned home to Milton to watch the afternoon baseball game on television and passed the evening, as was his custom, with his poker gang. He died suddenly the next morning while he was preparing to depart for the annual meeting of the Medical Library Association in Milwaukee. He was seventy-six.

"Jim Ballard was an unusual person," eulogized Henry Viets with his usual understatement in *The New England Journal of Medicine*:

He presumably knew more about old medical books than almost anyone living in his time. . . He was meticulous in the care of the valuable material entrusted to him, although careless about his personal appearance and often a little gruff in manner. When it came to the treasures in the Library, no one could have been a better custodian and guarded them more carefully, or handled them with more reverence. He came to symbolize the Library and ran it, of course, as a "one man show" long after it might have become more standardized in form. He was what the book world would call a "unicum," one of a kind, who set a pattern that can never be duplicated.

Mr. Ballard's life spanned a long period, and he was fond of recalling the time when he delivered books to Oliver Wendell Holmes in the last part of the nineteenth century. Harvey Cushing, William Osler, Arnold Klebs, Richard Cabot and a host of other Boston physicians knew him intimately and, indeed, were his close friends. He had the happy faculty of getting along in all walks of life and was equally at home in a bookseller's dusty warehouse in Paris or Madrid and in the more stately confines of some of the Back Bay physicians' houses. He was always a little reserved and perhaps difficult to know well, but once the bridge was crossed, no one could have a finer friend or one with more enduring qualities.[37]

"If many had modeled their ideals and practices on his," mused McDaniel from his more distant vantage, "he would scarcely have retained to the end the unique position that was, and will remain, his. A unique position is potentially, of course, a lonely one. One is happy to think that that was not the case with our dean, who, nowhere a stranger, built also his own little world largely with his own hands, dwelt in it contentedly, and left it, finally, full of years and honors. The loneliness, it so happens, is ours."[38]

In the rush of repairs and renovations which had overtaken the Boston Medical Library as it was caught up and swept along by the waves of the success of its efforts "to create out of whole cloth a giving constituency which does not now exist," the quaint old Victorian rocking chair of the founding president had been spotted among the memories of his presence in Holmes Hall and sent off by some enthusiast to the upholsterer. One morning not long after its return, the frayed and faded fabric so well worn by the Holmesian backsides replaced with the whole cloth of the new constituency, a note was discovered in the seat, directed to the trustees. They inserted it in their minutes, and their silence was almost sorrowful:[39]

Dear Trustee
If you were curator of the Sistine Chapel, would you dare to reupholster Michaelangelo's vaults? Or would you like it if someone took a notion to send your head off to be reupholstered just because a few cracks had developed in it! Spare, do spare the grim touch of modernism in our Holmes corner.
A. Reader

11

Love's Labour's Retrieved

1955 · 1960

The year 1955 produced striking grounds for hope that the Boston Medical Library, at eighty, had secured a new lease not alone on 8 The Fenway, but on life. In the short term, the endeavors of its custodians to mend fences, influence neighbors and win more friends had paid off beyond expectation. More than enough had been raised ($316,115 in pledges, 98.5 per cent honored, when the books were closed on the Greater Service Campaign in 1957) to put the house in reasonable order and to stack the void, at least until the centennial. After that not-so-distant day the onus would be another generation's. . . perhaps by then the outpouring would be miniaturized on microfilm or memorized by a mechanical brain.

Never had the membership been so large (238 succumbed to the evangelism of Secretary Richard Warren, raising the current roll to 1156), or so convivial (the first annual dinner meeting at the Harvard Club on April 6 attracted the greatest gathering since 1911). Seized with the fervor of the convert, the trustees cast off the bushel altogether and engaged Everett R. Spencer, Jr., the effectively low-key Director of Public Relations and Administration for the Medical Society next door, to nurse the candle's flame as their own part-time advance man. His calm persuasions over the next decade swelled the fellowship to 1446.

One void had hardly been filled when another was created by the death of Director Ballard in May, ripe in years and service beyond the allotted span. With him passed an epoch, measured in its pace, and now modernism, grim of touch, was in the coachman's seat. Overdue, some said. But in the meanwhile, the patient succedaneum-apparent, Assistant Charles Colby, had been lured away to the University of Missouri as Chief Medical Librarian in September of 1954, with the bonus of the assistant professorship of medical bibliography a year later. The trustees appointed Henry Viets acting director and asked Richard Warren, who had been succeeded as secretary by Franz J. Ingelfinger at the 1955 annual meeting, to head a committee to replace Mr. Ballard. It had not far to look. Mr. Colby was induced to return with the title of Librarian, full time, conferred by the same amendment to the by-laws at the 1956 meeting which eliminated the position of Director and created that of Curator, to which Dr. Viets was appointed. Librarian Colby returned to The Fenway on April 2, 1956.

Further vital signs of recovery in 1955 were a ruddy flush brought on by an unexpected succession of financial transfusions, and a pulse quickened by the prospect of more to come in positively immeasurable volume.

The first step, as it frequently does, involved a course of antihemorrhagic action and was prescribed by President Allen in 1953 with the suggestion that the Medical Society write off over a period of years the $19,000 balance of the interest-bearing loan of $23,703 it had advanced to the Library in 1931 as its share of the 1929 fund drive. In 1955 the Society forgave $2000 of this obligation and after a suspenseful pause of a few years erased the remainder entirely.

After the Director's death Dr. George Cheever Shattuck offered to catalyze a James F. Ballard Fund with $5000 contingent upon the raising of another $20,000, the income to be used for staff salaries and pensions, or if not needed for that purpose, as free endowment. By the end of 1958 the Ballard Fund stood at $29,000, a generous reserve but far short of the financing of a staff retirement program, which was deferred by the trustees indefinitely.

As recognition, and stimulus, the board approved the display of a plaque bearing the names of those in whose memory the Library had received $5000 or more, including James Bourne Ayer, Lincoln Davis, Henry Lyman, George Howard Monks, Edward H. Bradford, Marius N. Smith-Petersen, Hugh Williams, James F. Ballard and Frank Howard Lahey. Dr. Lahey had died in June 27, 1953, six years after his Clinic began paying for a professional membership and for the fellowships of his staff, which in 1947 came to $845. The Lahey group got up a fund to finish off the periodical room in his memory, and it was dedicated on September 12, 1956.

Two substantial gifts came to the Library in 1955 by the hands of third parties. The late Mabel H. Ricker of Lynn was the source of about $20,000; her attorney had enjoyed the privileges of Holmes Hall and suggested she include the BML in her will, and she did. The other unsought benefaction was a distribution of $83,320 from the residual estate of David Nevins, who died in 1898 leaving about $900,000 in trust to his wife and daughter. This surviving child, Mrs. William F. Morgan, died in 1954, when the estate, under the careful cultivation of Boston trusteedom, had grown to nearly two million dollars. Mrs. Morgan's husband, one of its trustees, struck upon the happy thought that the residue of $1,666,410 could be nicely divided among twenty charities, and it was his physician, a Fellow of the Boston Medical Library, who whispered in Mr. Morgan's ear with such excellent effect.

By far the best news of the year, and the most sensational of the century, was not of a gift but of the intimation of one never approached in the history of the Library, in magnitude or in mystery. It all began, or rather surfaced, with the receipt of a copy of the will of Dennistoun M. Bell of New York, who died on December 16, 1954. His estate was divided into two parts, of which one fourth of one was to revert to the Boston Medical Library on the death of his widow, and possibly a fourth of the other at her discretion. It appeared that this might come to as much as $400,000, or even twice that if Mrs. Bell should ever feel so inclined.

Very little was known in Boston of this unaccountably and uncommonly generous friend of the Library. He was not a Fellow, and although he represented himself and was addressed as "Doctor Bell," his name had never appeared in the *American Medical Directory* of the American Medical Association as a physician licensed to practice in the United States. Not for fourteen years after Bell's death did Henry Viets, the only surviving figure at the Library who had had any contact with him, spread anything at all upon the record. The occasion was the trustees' meeting on March 19, 1969, a few month's after Mrs. Bell's demise:

> Evidence that he actually held an M.D. degree cannot be found. He prepared and sold an anti-acid remedy about 1899. In 1907 the name of his product was changed to Bel-Ans and it is still being sold widely. At about 1950 Dr. Bell appeared at the Boston Medical Library and was a very pleasant, tall Scot who sought a complete collection of the Cabot Case records. Mr. Ballard assembled and had bound for him a complete set of these from 1915 to 1949. This set which Dr. Bell ultimately returned to the Library is one of the few sets of these case records in existence. They provide a unique indication of clinical advances in this 35 year period. Dr. Bell often entertained Dr. Viets and Mr. Ballard at luncheon at the Ritz Hotel. He retired to his large estate in Amagansett, Long Island, and on his decease, December 16, 1954, his age was recorded in the New York Times as 75. Prior to his death, Dr. Arthur Allen, then President of the BML, visited him in New York and persuaded him to remember the BML in his will.

Dennistoun Bell's return of the bound Case Records of the MGH from *The New England Journal of Medicine* in 1951, as Dr. Viets correctly recalled, was recorded in that year's annual report; a bibliographic contribution in 1952 was attributed to him but not described. Any officer of the Library so caviling as to inquire further into the background of its enigmatic benefactor could have learned that four of the principal products of his firm, Bell and Company, manufacturing chemists, had been blacklisted for many years by the Council on Pharmacy and Chemistry of the American Medical Association in its annual publication, *New and Nonofficial Remedies*, a mark of recognition not accorded even Mrs. Pinkham's compound. In 1953, in fact—the year before Bell's death and the last in which the "Bibliography of Unaccepted Products" was included in *Remedies*—"Bell-ans," "Salacetin," "Sal-Codeia" and "Cascarans" were still among the ostracized.[1]

In 1905 the Council had assayed "Salacetin," found its ingredients to be something less than described on the package (mainly sodium bicarbonate and acetanilid) and warned of toxic side effects from its uncontrolled over-the-counter distribution; nor was the Council any less concerned over the addition of codeine to make of it "Sal-Codeia."[2] "Pa-pay-ans, Bell" tablets were introduced to the public around the turn of the century by way of medical journals and naive physicians. In 1909 the Council tested this cure-all for indigestion, peritonitis, cholera morbus, seasickness, vertigo and what have you along that line which claimed to contain the enzyme papain as a digestant; it isolated sodium bicarbonate and charcoal, but no sign of papain, and refused the product recognition with the comment: "Pa-pay-ans (Bell) seems to be consistently fulfilling the life history of the average nostrum. Made of well-known drugs and invested by its manufacturers—or exploiters—with virtues absurdly disproportionate to the known properties of the alleged constituents of the nostrum, the preparation was introduced to the world *via* the medical profession. With the help of thoughtless physicians, aided by a skillful and aggressive advertising campaign and augmented by the 'free sample' device, the business grew and prospered. . ."[3]

Dennistoun Bell's company in 1914 notified physicians that "Pa-pay-ans, Bell" would henceforth be "Bell-ans" as "shorter, pleasanter sounding and better." Commented the Council: "Bell & Co. are changing a misleading name into a meaningless one."[4] Three years later "Bell-ans" was being advertised in the lay press as a remedy that "Absolutely Removes Indigestion," and the hounds of the AMA were back on the scent.

"S. Q. Lapius, M.D." wrote a lengthy report for the Council in the AMA's *Journal* observing that the name change "was probably not made entirely for euphonious reasons, as alleged, especially when one considers that the name of a nostrum is its most valuable asset. It is much more likely that as analyses indicate there was not and probably never had been any papain present in the product, the name was changed for fear that some day the misleading term 'Pa-pay-ans' might bring the preparation in conflict with the federal Food and Drugs Act." If it was even approximately true that 100,000 American physicians prescribed "Bell-ans," as the manufacturers claimed, "Dr. Lapius" added, "it is a serious reflection on the medical profession, for the Council examined Bell-ans and reported its findings nearly eight years ago. . . and the statements made in that report are as incontrovertible today as they were then."[5]

In the 1921 edition of *Nostrums and Quackery* the AMA put it on the line: "The whole secret of the commercial success of Bell-ans lies in the mystery of its composition and the fake and misleading claims that have been made for it. The same tablets put out under a non-proprietary name, as an open formula and with claims that were reasonable and true, would have had practically no sale."[6]

Thus by a tithe upon his gullibility was the American consumer relieved of his loose change (and, one hopes, of some digestive distress in the bargain) for the advancement of medical bibliography, while Dennistoun Bell, by the exacting of it, cast from his conscience the long-standing indebtedness he evidently felt toward the legion of unthinking physicians whom he adopted as brethren and who had helped his business to grow and indeed to prosper.

Dr. Allen's initiative and charm in securing the assurance of a piece of this wonderfully profitable anti-acid action and his many other achievements in behalf of the Boston Medical Library moved Dr. Grant V. Rodkey and various professional associates and friends to establish in 1956 the Dr. Arthur W. Allen Restoration Fund for the improvement of the facilities; by the year's end 270 of them had given $15,700. On March 15, 1958 Arthur Allen died in Boston. He was seventy, rounding out his second three-year term of a presidency during which he inspired a resurgence of appreciation of the Boston Medical Library which generated new highs in membership, the funds to complete the stack addition and an inflow of financial support culminating in the promise of a bequest that would dwarf anything ever received.

At the annual meeting in April 1958, a few days after the deaths of Dr. Allen and of his own wife, Lucy, a week earlier on March 7, Howard B. Sprague was elected President. Dr. Walter S. Burrage, son of the late secretary, replaced him as treasurer, and Dr. Earle M. Chapman succeeded Dr. Ingelfinger as secretary. At their first meeting the trustees re-elected Dr. Garland assistant treasurer and added the vice presidency.

Sprague was sixty-two, a graduate of Harvard College, and of the Medical School in 1922. His career in cardiology had been spent at the MGH with Dr. Paul D. White. He was the first of White's residents to join the medical staff, from which he retired to the Board of Consultation in 1956, the year of his appointment as a lecturer in medicine at Harvard. He had been chief of staff at the House of the Good Samaritan and served as a captain in the Navy medical corps in the Pacific during World War II. Dr. Sprague's contributions to cardiology were many, from the Sprague-Bowles stethoscope to the promotion of national and international lay-medical cooperation in the study and treatment of heart disease. He was a realist and a caustic wit, two qualities which he would draw on abundantly during the next two years.

Ironically, but perhaps not too bitterly so, those heroic remedies of 1955 proved out as but palliative. The Greater Service Program from its inception had been a calculated risk venture. It is axiomatically easier and more glamorous to raise money for such tangibles as bricks, mortar and stacks than for endowment from which to pay salaries, purchase fuel and replace light bulbs. The first phase succeeded in renewing the storage capacity of the Library for another score of years (it was supposed) and had enough reserve impetus to bring in more than $100,000 of the endowment of $750,000 sought before it ran out of steam. The anxiously anticipated Bell bequest, however, would not be released until his widow's death and as late as 1959 was not expected to exceed half a million dollars. Still a bird in the bush.

In hand, it took merely five years for inflation and the upward push on operating costs from vastly increased demands for service to nullify the substantial additional income produced by the alliance with the Massachusetts Medical Society and the extremely successful recruitment of independent Fellows. The disconsolate trustees faced a projected deficit of $15,000 for 1957, and no relief in sight.

Under the circumstances they were less than elated by the word which had filtered across the Fens that Harvard was talking seriously about building a brand new medical library from the ground up which could hardly help but overshadow, if not wither, their own. The first mention of such a ghastly possibility is in the trustees' minutes of March 20, 1957, when Joseph Garland wondered if such a talked-of behemoth installed a mile away might not diminish the need for the Boston Medical Library and impair its traditional functions. He and the other trustees were assured by Sidney Burwell (who had passed the deanship to Dr. George Packer Berry in 1949 and had in fact been building this library in the sky with him and the committee on library, of which he was chairman, at least since 1954) that no whetting of rivalries whatsoever was intended, that Harvard was duly considering her sister medical libraries and even had in mind sharing some sort of storage system with her friends on The Fenway. Harvard's plans in reality could not have struck as a thunderbolt upon the BML, which already was sharing in one phase of the School's concern with the reorganization of its ever less satisfactory library through an interlibrary committee that for a year had been trying to synchronize the accession and general availability of medical books and journals in the Boston area. Neither was it a secret that the Medical School had set out in 1956 to raise $58,000,000 over a decade which overlapped by four years the College's staggering campaign for $82,500,000, or that a new library was among the objectives of the Harvard Medical Fund.

The realization that his reach might at long last be within grasping distance of the great library which was at the core of his vision of the Medical School of the future really dawned on Dean Berry not very long after the death of Francis A. Countway, the retired president of Lever Brothers' American branch, in September 1955.

Countway was a tycoon *á la soap opèra bouffe*. When he was sixteen he dropped out of Somerville High School to take a job as bookkeeper for a local molasses dealer who owned a side interest in Curtis, Davis & Company, makers of Welcome soap in East Cambridge. From that moment it was the American dream come true in the sudsiest tradition. The young fellow hit the road selling Welcome soap so slickly that fourteen years after William Lever (who had started almost as humbly in England) bought Curtis, Davis in 1913, Countway was elevated to the presidency of the Lever brothers' American operation, at the age of thirty-seven. The expansion of the colonial offshoot under the regency of the Yankee supersalesman is a frothy chapter in the history of advertising and marketing. "Nine out of ten screen stars use Lux," was the word from Countway, and his countrywomen flocked to buy. In 1939 there was enough left over to reward him for this and other similar indispensable pieces of cosmetic advice with a salary of $469,713, exceeded only by the gross take of that other dream merchant from across the continent, Louis B. Mayer. The same year, in tribute to cleanliness (and out of gratitude to its antonym), Countway built a shining new office building on Memorial Drive in Cambridge.

"The Chief" acquired a Dusenberg and a set of golf clubs. At the end of one hot day on the links he was inspired (it is said) by the effects of Lifebuoy soap, another of his products, to juxtapose the initials "B.O." by which his publicists drummed the shame of body odor into the semiconsciousness of a sweaty and soap-mad public. The man was the personally unprepossessing master of the grand gesture. His every whim was the command of his "fixers," who when none were claimed to be available hired private railroad cars, swept the occupants from royal hotel suites and bought up blocks of sold-out first-night tickets for the delectation of the impressionable. So mighty was he in his own commercial seat (and such a deliverer of the goods) that on one occasion Lever's American president is reported to have shut down all production in the plant to insure absolute silence while he recorded a speech to be sent over for replay at a board meeting in Britain. Countway was not famous for his charities though he was said to have helped a number of boys through college. It is obvious that he was gifted with an overpowering will in his singleminded pursuit, that he was a shrewd judge of executive talent, a brilliant opportunist, an early virtuoso at manipulation of the mass media and positively clairvoyant in his instinct for exploiting the simplistic in the American self-image. When Countway retired in 1946 Lord Leverhulme (William Lever's son) observed with satisfaction that in his American agent's thirty-three years at the top he had increased annual sales from $600,000 to $200,000,000.[8]

Mr. Countway's life companion was his unmarried sister Sanda (for Gussanda, although her given name was Edith), who kept house for her bachelor brother after 1927 at Longwood Towers in Brookline. For a few years following her graduation from Jackson College in 1904 Miss Countway taught Latin in Chelsea Senior High School. A former pupil remembered her as "a powerhouse of knowledge. She brought to her Latin class each day new ideas on Caesar's Gallic Wars, her animation making the text a living topic. . . A truly beautiful person, she had a cameo face, slightly olive in complexion, high cheekbones with a touch of pink. The eyes were a liquid brown. Her hair was chestnut, framing her face and brushed over the 'rat' foundation women wore in those days. Hers was a spritelike figure, small and energetic, moving at all times, never allowing boredom. She drove a Ford two-seater each day from Somerville in those days when cars were rare and a woman at the wheel even more so. . . Teaching seemed to be her one ambition. . . Like her brother, she had her potentialities, but in the limited confines of a four-walled schoolroom."[9]

Francis A. Countway died on September 19, 1955 at seventy-nine. He left about $6,000,000 in trust, a quarter of the net income to his brother George, the balance to sister Sanda along with the power to dispose of the principal by her will. He designated Miss Countway and the Old Colony Trust Company his trustees. Countway admired the bank's chairman, Robert Cutler, who for many years had a large part in the affairs of the Peter Bent Brigham Hospital and the Harvard Medical School, as had his brother, Dr. Elliott C. Cutler, who died in 1947. Mr. Cutler and Dean Berry persuaded Miss Countway that a new library for the Medical School would be the ideal memorial to Francis, who (it was said) had been interested in the advancement of science. (Well, he *did* enroll Lever Brothers as the first nonmedical professional member of the Boston Medical Library in 1934, a mode of advancement which terminated with his retirement and the elevation of Charles Luckman, which was followed in three years by the firm's removal to New York City and Luckman's removal from the firm.)

George Countway, the surviving brother, died on January 8, 1958. Soon after, Dr. Berry brought Ralph T. Esterquest to the Medical School as Librarian to succeed the retiring Miss Anna Holt. Esterquest was a genial Chicagoan of forty-six, a graduate of Northwestern University and widely known as a frontiersman in the science (and art) of the new librarianship. His reputation was based largely on his achievements in interlibrary cooperation as the first director of the Midwest Inter-Library Center (later the Center for Research Libraries) in Chicago, wherein sixteen universities set up a common depository for their less-used collections to make room for current publications in their own libraries. The Dean was entirely aware of Mr. Esterquest's "extraordinary capacity to bring library services into complementary and supplementary partnership," as he considerately couched it seven years later when that "partnership" had become a reality.[10]

George Countway's death accelerated events. On April 1 Dr. Burwell addressed the annual meeting of the Boston Medical Library at which Howard Sprague was elected to fill out the unexpired term of Arthur Allen. His subject was the School's library plans.[11] As with the trustees a year previously, Burwell was at some pains to reassure the members that Harvard had no desire to preempt the local medical library scene, that cooperation and collaboration were its aims in order to minimize duplication while building up the greatly enlarged core collection which the explosion of the biological sciences demanded, and pooling with the other libraries less-used material. He suggested that the Union Catalogue be extended to include the journal holdings of the Boston University and Tufts University medical libraries, with the BML as the information center. And then Dr. Burwell dramatically parted the curtain for a peak at the perimeter of George Berry's vision: a Harvard Medical Library with double the book capacity, double the staff, triple the reader capacity and triple the budget. Cost: give or take eight million dollars. "Dean Berry tells me that these funds will be found."

Sanda Countway was anxious to see her brother memorialized while she was alive. On June 16 her advisers established the Countway Charitable Foundation, to which she assigned all her rights in his estate save for her life income. By this means she assured the Harvard Medical School $3,500,000 toward construction of its library, a million dollars for the central building of the Boston Museum of Science and half a million for the Boys' Clubs of Boston.

With this egg in the nest, Dean Berry, Dr. Burwell, Mr. Esterquest and University Librarian Douglas W. Bryant got down to the serious business of planning and on October 15, 1958 produced a prospectus entitled "Program for a New Library Building to Serve the Harvard Medical Center—Preliminary Edition Circulated for Criticism." Copies were given the BML trustees for their meeting on November 19.

The planners conceived of Harvard's first separately housed medical library in the light of two trends: the integration of the social and behavioral sciences into medical education, and the realization that the walls between the specialties had to be breeched if there was going to be a freer exchange of ideas. If it could advance the latter objective, they prophesied, "it will earn its place in the history of medical education and in the development of comprehensive medicine itself." Dissemination was to have overwhelming priority over conservation. The library would not be a storehouse; the least used books would be put away somewhere else. The interior design would be flexible to shifting emphases on educational material and techniques but aimed above all at making it as painless as could be for seeker to find the sought-for. With manifest pleasure the planners banished from beneath this neo-epicurean plane tree of medical learning every marbled reminder, every musty remnant, every stiff-backed shred of Shattuck Street (and Fenway) Puritanism:

> Hopefully, it may provide the quality of relaxation that a man finds when he goes fishing, leaving the noise and pressures of the city behind and immersing himself in the stillness and beauty of the countryside. . . Although the Library cannot supply a trout stream, it should be able to provide a setting that gives repose to the harried spirit. . . In spite of the misgivings of most of us, the evidence is striking that many people work more comfortably with music. The Library should be completely wired and equipped for piped-in music. . . but control switches should make it possible to include or exclude any area at will so that no one is forced to be part of a captive audience.

The Francis A. Countway Library of Medicine, according to the most educated estimates of 1958, should have a capacity of 389,500 volumes, in contrast to the stock in Building A of 106,775 (an increase from double to triple since Dr. Burwell's April projection), and 1000 current unbound periodicals on display. Esterquest could find no suitable formula for the number of reader accommodations but settled on 740, a triple expansion. Beyond those associated with the Medical School and its affiliates, access was to be limited to those qualifying in the following categories, of which the first and the last only would have the borrowing privilege:

a. Serious research workers from other parts of Harvard (e.g., Chemistry faculty, Biology Ph.D. candidate) who need to examine literature available in Library.
b. Serious research workers, not Harvard-associated. Needs are similar.
c. Students. Harvard-associated and others. Permitted to be "readers" only if material they properly need cannot be had in their "own" library. Use is occasional, of short duration.
d. Doctors and professional persons not attached to any school are occasional users. Rarely search literature at depth.
e. Others, not normally encouraged to use the Library, may occasionally become a "reader" for a brief period if his need is quickly and easily satisfied.
f. Library staff readers.

The "Building Program" defined as its final aspiration "a library service that is correlated with other libraries in the area; inter-library cooperation must have a chance to bring access to increased resources." Nowhere did it mention the Boston Medical Library.

After forty years that gadfly prophet, Professor Frederic Lewis, was on the point of honor. His balloon of 1921 had collapsed with that scornful pin prick of Farlow's: "What does Harvard have to offer?" The worm had turned, the shoe was on the other foot, the coin had been reversed. Now the Medical School was sitting on three and a half millions of Countway money, and $1,400,000 for endowment from Harold S. Vanderbilt, and $200,000 from the Markle Foundation. . . while down the Muddy River the Boston Medical Library, having gone for broke to fill its last void with stacks, faltered toward spatial and financial exhaustion.

Officially, Harvard offered nothing. But from the Dean's office the bait was dangled: a spacious new home, and financial security. The catch: the third largest medical library in America. The trustees could not conceal their interest.

On December 9, 1958 Sprague, Viets, Chapman and Colby met with Burwell and Esterquest at the Medical School. The President of the Boston Medical Library frankly proposed a marriage, to which the Harvard side responded encouragingly. An informal suit was at once begun and continued through the holidays into January, when on the fifteenth a cautionary ensign was run up the masthead of *The New England Journal of Medicine* by Editor Garland, alerting the fellows of the Massachusetts Medical Society and of the Library (of which he was vice president) that a matter of consequence was under discussion:

> Of almost equal importance to the physical and moral support of the Boston Medical Library is the necessity of a realistic appraisal of its place and function in relation to the new bibliothecal center that the Harvard Medical School is soon to erect a short and pleasant mile away, across the Fenway. It may not be entirely enough for any predetermined role, such as that of serving the practicing profession, to be relegated, however graciously, to the Boston Medical Library, or at least not until the use of such a library by practicing physicians has been appraised.
>
> It is necessary for the protection of the Library's financial investment and for the Society's interest in it, as well as for the indispensable part that the Library has played and continues to play in the medical life of the area, that the two institutions work out, in practical detail, an inter-related and complementary position in the medical community for each. In this way a costly duplication of resources and a still more costly dispersion of interests will be avoided. It must still be remembered that a free public medical library serves its area in ways that a university library can hardly be expected to match.[12]

The day after the publication of this editorial caution a committee of the trustees consisting of Bradford, Rodkey and Lamar Soutter, Associate Dean of the Boston University School of Medicine, met to worry about the Library's financial future. Their report six days later was glum.[13] Since the wind-up of the Greater Service Program campaign, the Ballard and Allen funds had accumulated totals of $29,000 and $33,000, to which had been added contributions of $4700 to "The Library Fund" initiated by a letter appeal from Secretary Chapman; $9500 as the fruit of Everett Spencer's labors; $16,000 in bequests, including an unrestricted one of $5000 from the estate of Dr. Joseph H. Pratt; $15,000 in response to a brochure, "Projects for Progress;" and $25,000 in grants from the Massachusetts Heart Association to endow the purchase of cardiovascular literature, obtained by Dr. Sprague and his colleagues. It all came to $132,000. Of course there was the Bell bequest somewhere in the offing.

Across the ledger from these contributions, all non-recurring except possibly for the Heart Fund's, was the critical need to overcome the $15,000 deficit, the pressing need for a $5000 annual employee insurance and retirement program, and the urgent need to spend at least another $25,000 to enlarge services by enlarging staff, to increase mail and delivery circulation and to maintain accessions. How and where was another $40,000 a year to be found? "Although this is a challenging figure," the committee reflected gloomily, "it does not seem advisable at the present time to attempt another 'high pressure' fund raising campaign. We do not want to enter the field just now as competitors with Harvard University; and furthermore, our past campaign occurred too recently to make the prospects of the repetition so soon afterwards at all favorable. The Library's problem, therefore, is where to seek funds by low pressure methods."

Various possibilities, mainly the suggestion that a publicity campaign of eighteen months or so might induce the Medical Society members to pay another dollar a year, were examined, none hopefully.

From this confrontation with financial reality, Sprague, Chapman, Garland and Colby turned to a second joint expedition into greener pastures with Berry, Burwell, Esterquest and Bryant at the Harvard Club on January 22. The Harvard delegation brought along "A Statement of Principles for Guidance in the Exploration of a Possible Collaborative Library Service by The Boston Medical Library and the Harvard Medical Library." This first open and unequivocal proposal for the formal alliance of the two libraries under one roof was unsigned but probably written by Ralph Esterquest. It was given close study, discussion, revision and legal examination and emerged under date of February 3, 1959, marked *confidential*, for the consideration of the respective governing bodies.

A. *Background and Purpose*

During recent years it has become increasingly apparent that the independent operation of two large medical libraries in Boston is inefficient and uneconomical. Both the Boston Medical Library and the Harvard Medical Library are being called upon to perform services that are increasingly similar. Both libraries are finding it necessary to collect and house large stocks of books and journals (the term "books," hereafter, is intended to include books, journals, manuscripts, and other library materials) that, to an increasing degree, duplicate each other. Efforts to coordinate collecting programs and services to avoid this duplication are thwarted by the practical realities of their locations: they are too far apart for easy walking, and the lack of parking space makes driving almost impossible. In short, busy doctors and research specialists are finding it more and more difficult to travel back and forth between the two libraries, using certain materials in one and other materials in the other.

The Boston Medical Library is handicapped in its service efforts by its obsolescent building. Its base and opportunities for financial support are inadequate for the task imposed by modern research demands. Its future appears to be a choice between a series of crisis-inspired financial drives or a progressive retrenching of services. Unmistakably, this trend has already begun.

More than a mile away—too far for ready mutual access—the Harvard Medical Library stands also at a cross-roads. It has outgrown its quarters, and its resources and its services are far below those which should be expected of a library serving the broad teaching and research program of the Harvard medical community. The growth of its collections has been deliberately limited in the past because the Boston Medical Library was in the city. This policy may have been a wise one in days gone by, but the scope of medical research, the proliferation of medical literature, the increasing dependence on libraries, and the enormous growth in numbers of the Harvard medical faculty and associated research personnel have made highly unrealistic any major dependence upon another library. The problem is intensified by the fact that whole new areas of knowledge are now becoming germane to medical research—areas which in the past were considered beyond the scope of a medical library. The formation of the Harvard Medical Center has been a further step that has made it mandatory that Harvard have at its heart its own first-class medical library. Fortunately, a generous gift has assured the construction of a proper medical library building, and other gifts will make possible the development of top-quality library resources, with appropriate service.

These events have brought into sharp focus the present and future relationships between these two libraries. The Boston Medical Library has extensive collections that could make a much greater contribution to medical research in the Commonwealth if its building and financial problems could be solved. The Harvard library is in the process of solving building and financial problems, and must begin now to collect further books and journals to meet its growing responsibilities. If present circumstances continue, many of these books and journals will duplicate materials in which the Boston Medical Library has already invested.

The evidence is clear that the interests of both libraries and the interests of the medical community would be better served if a way could be found for bringing the two libraries into some kind of collaborative operation in a single, well-functioning, modern building.

It is proposed, therefore, that the Governing Boards of Harvard and of Boston Medical Library entertain proposals for a collaborative effort between the two libraries along the lines of the following outline, having regard to the terms upon which the respective libraries and their supporting endowments are held and to all other considerations relevant to these proposals.

It is proposed that such a collaborative library facility be organized and operated in a manner most appropriate to the common end: adequate resources and services in support of medical practice, medical teaching, and medical research in the community as a whole.

It is proposed that Harvard furnish land and construct a library building to house the collaborative operation, that the Boston Medical Library dispose of its land and building, and that book collections, personnel, and services of both libraries be combined into a library service of maximum usefulness to the community.

B. *Organization and Operations*

1. *Primary Objective.* A library exists to serve readers. The collaborative library operation of the Harvard Medical School and the Boston Medical Library would be so constituted and so organized that it would serve with maximum effectiveness the individuals and groups that comprise its appropriate clientele. Good service depends upon comprehensive collections within the appropriate scope, easy and efficient access to the books, journals, and other library materials, comfortable and efficient reading space and facilities. Such considerations would be the determining criteria for the form of organization, the physical facilities, and the operating policies of the joint library service.

2. *Joint Sponsorship.* The agreement to operate a collaborative library service would not dissolve the independence of either party. Both the Board of Trustees of Boston Medical Library and the President and Fellows of Harvard College would continue to hold, manage and invest the endowments relating to their respective libraries and each would retain final authority over the disposition

and expenditure of its funds. Each would also retain title to its own books, periodicals and other items in its Library and would acquire title to all materials acquired in the future by the expenditure of its funds or by gift to it.

3. *A Single Operation.* Because service to readers is the primary objective, it would be the intent to operate a single, unified library, in a modern building, designed and constructed on functional principles. In order that readers would not be referred from one area or desk to another, the book stocks would be inter-filed on the shelves, or shelved in such areas as would be most effective in terms of reader convenience. The separate ownership of books and journals would be shown by suitable book-plates, identification, etc., but the reader would find material on his subject in one place, as convenience and appropriateness might dictate. Separate departments and reading rooms would be maintained as desirable in terms of service. For example, a history of medicine department, with outstanding resources of early books, and a special "physicians' reading room," with attractive furnishings, might be special BML features. A special students' room, students' conversation rooms, and an audio-visual department are examples of special Harvard features. Many other areas and features might be operated in common; for example: general periodical reading room, indexes and abstracts alcove, public card catalog, auditorium. The distribution and use of staff would also be in accordance with service to readers. The clientele would be defined as the total clientele of the two libraries, as the two governing bodies might from time to time designate.

4. *Executive Committee.* The Board of Trustees of the Boston Medical Library and the Harvard Medical School would each appoint four of its own members (including respectively the President and the Dean, serving *ex officio*), to an "Executive Committee of the Library" and would delegate general administrative authority to this Committee. The Executive Committee of the Library would elect one of its own members to serve as Chairman, for a one-year term, subject to re-election. The Executive Committee would meet regularly and be subject to call by either of the parent organizations, by three of its own members, or by the librarian. The librarian would serve as secretary of the Executive Committee.

5. *Fiscal Control.* Neither the Executive Committee nor the collaborative library service would hold property in its own right. Property could be held by either of the parent groups, and each would have final authority over its use and over the disbursement of its own funds. The adoption of the annual budget by both parent groups would, in effect, delegate authority for disbursing appropriated funds to the Executive Committee and the librarian.

6. *Name of Library Service.* The name of the collaborative library service might be:

THE COUNTWAY LIBRARY OF MEDICINE
Operated By
The Harvard Medical Library
The Boston Medical Library

C. *Proposed Resolution*

If the foregoing statement of principles is acceptable, it is proposed that the governing authorities adopt them and authorize the creation of a suitable joint

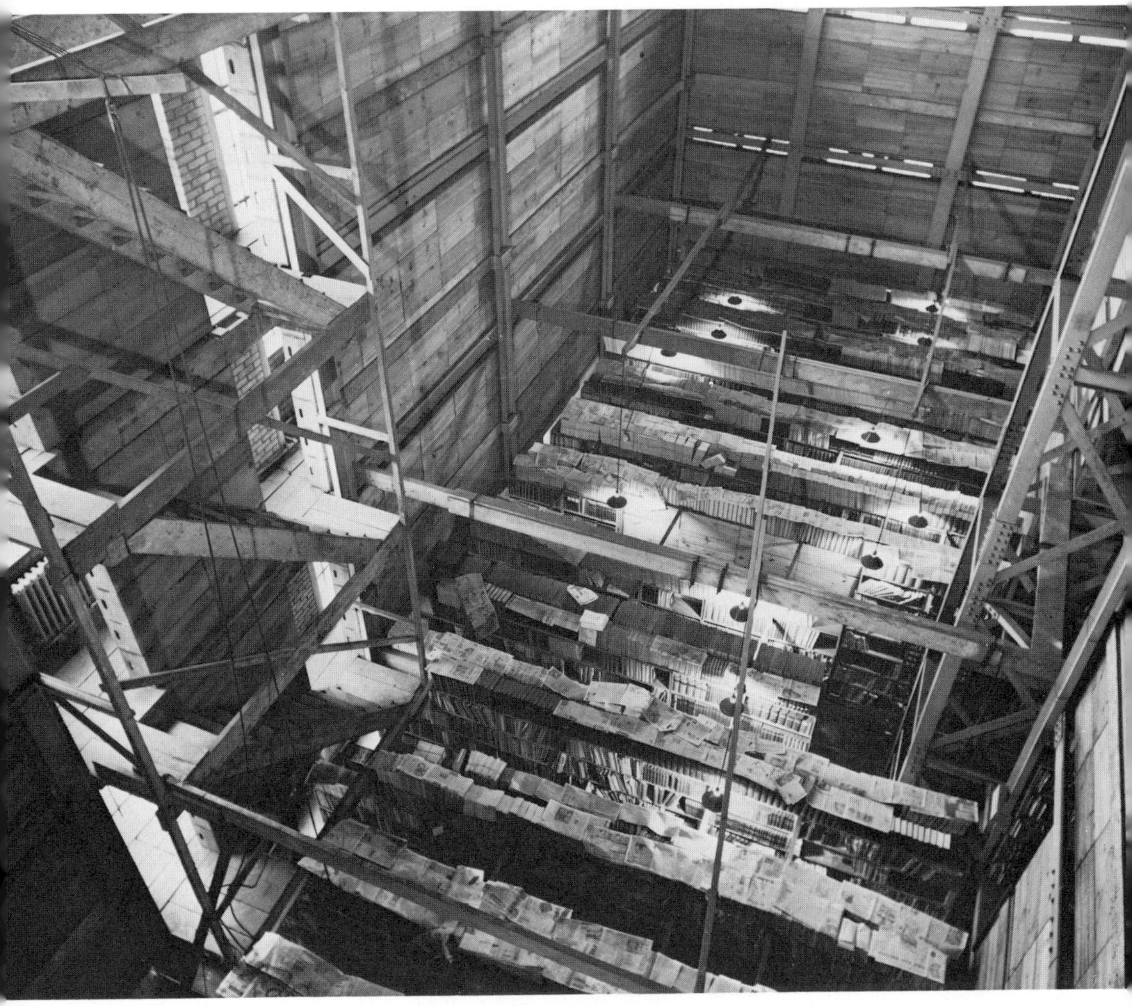

The Aching Void. A view of the incompleted stack addition, 1953

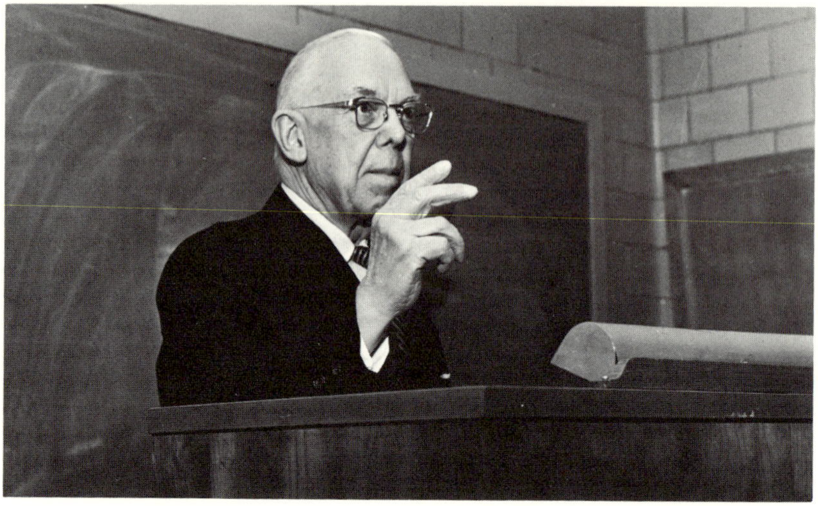

Henry R. Viets, M.D., 1963

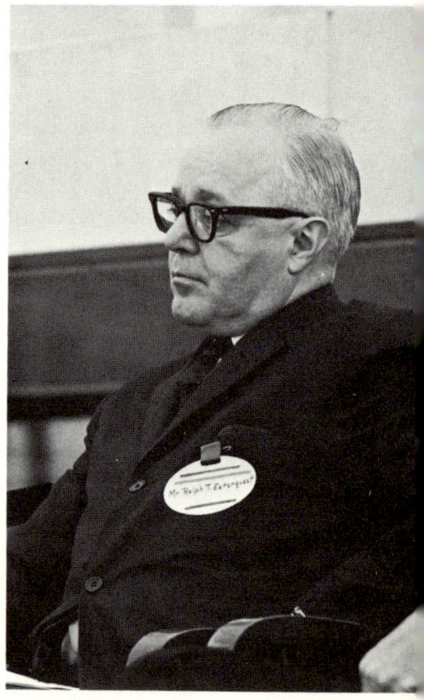

Ralph T. Esterquest, 1965

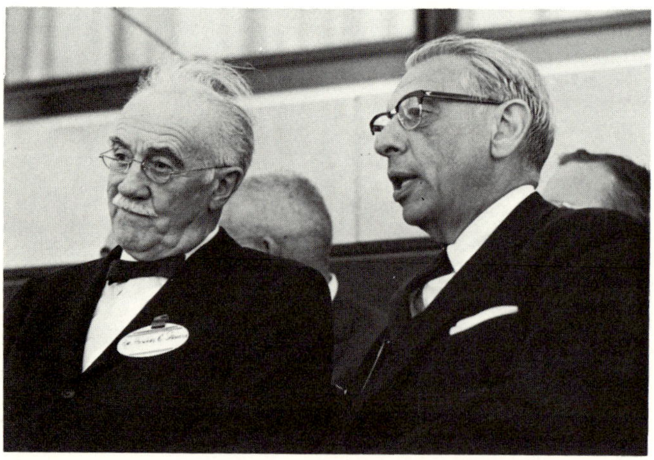

Howard B. Sprague, M.D., and George Packer Berry, M.D., 1965

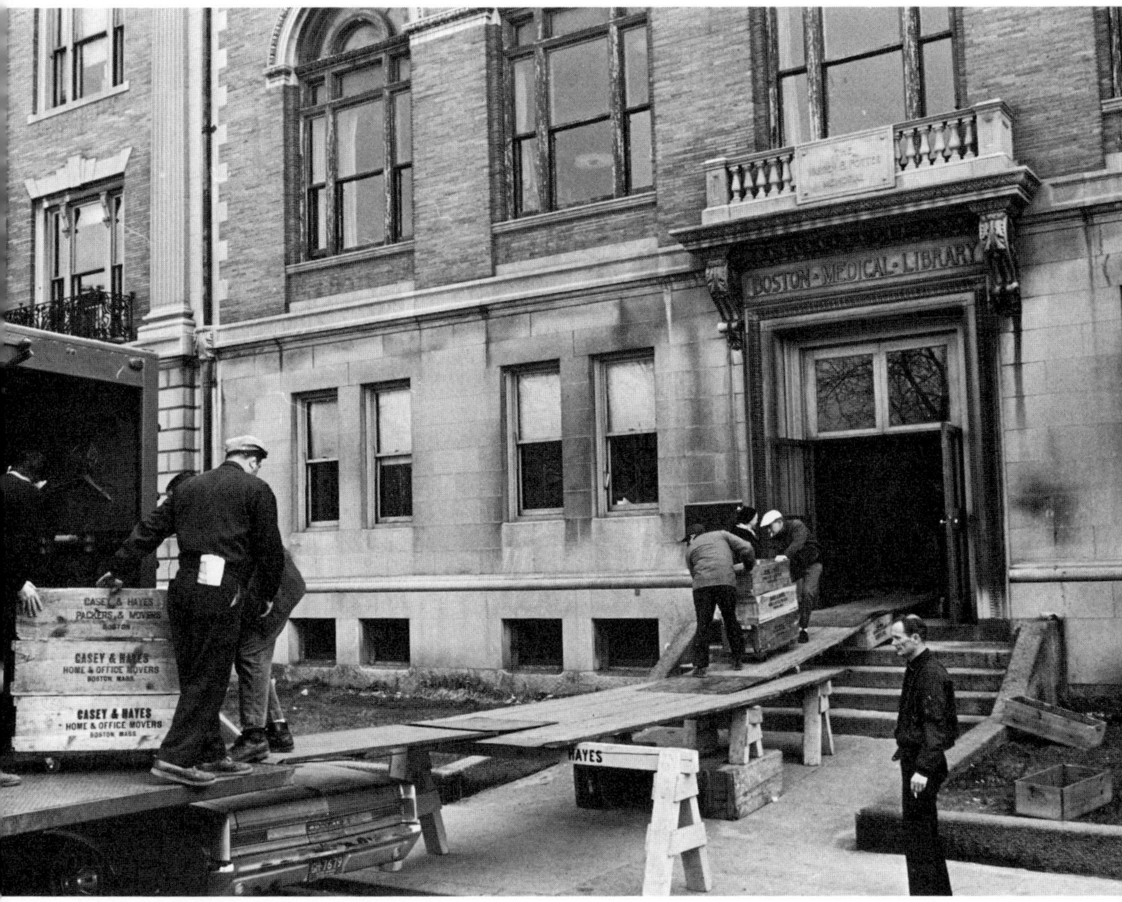

Moving out of 8 The Fenway, June 14, 1965

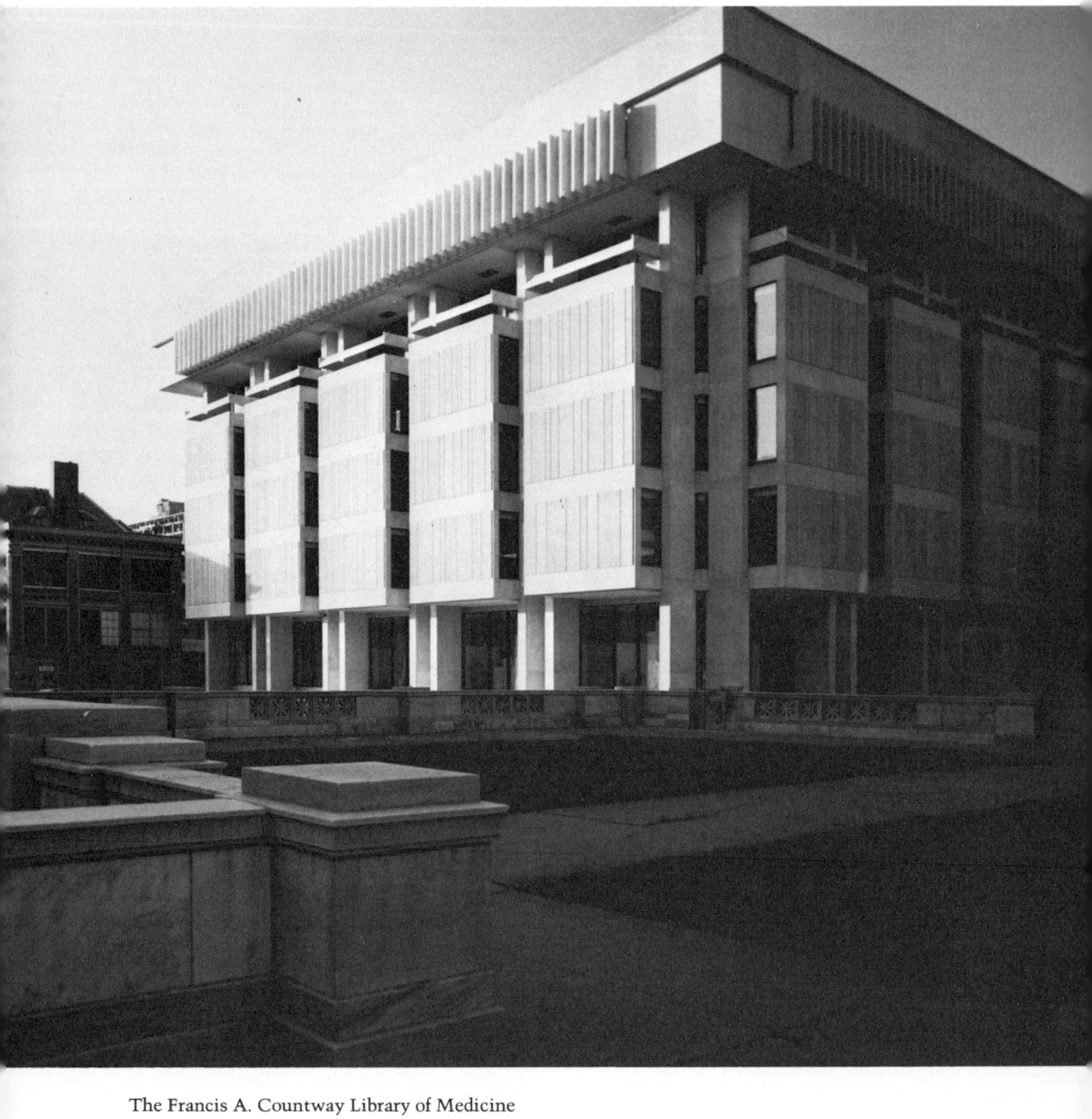

The Francis A. Countway Library of Medicine

committee to develop a detailed plan for collaborative library service, such plan to be subject to ratification by both parties.

The "Statement of Principles" was well received by nearly all the BML trustees present at their meeting on February 17, 1959, with President Sprague in the lead. All vigorously agreed that the bibliographic interests in the Boston University and Tufts medical schools, as well as any future schools,[14] the Massachusetts Medical Society and the profession at large, and indeed the public, must be protected, but whether the Harvard proposal provided adequate assurances on this score was a question which was viewed with varying degrees of skepticism. Dr. Joseph M. Hayman, Jr., the Tufts dean, personally favored the merger but said his faculty was opposed. Soutter led the opposition for the executive committee of the BU faculty with a strong expression of suspicion that Harvard would wind up in control of the Boston Medical Library as entirely as the whale swallowed Jonah, to which Chapman parried that "Jonah achieved immortality by a procedure without which Jonah would never have been heard again." Viets viewed the Harvard statement as a generous offer which threatened neither absorption nor liquidation, especially if the BML were to have its own wing. Garland approved in general but expressed reservations concerning protection of the interests of the other medical schools and the place of his *Journal.*

It was Charles Bradford who put his finger on the implicit stakes and hazards in what he saw as a "splendid concept [which] offers an ideal solution to the problems of the Boston Medical Library and promises to improve the existing medical library facilities of the community at large."[15] He warned that under no circumstances should the board enter into an agreement with Harvard which in any respect abridged the Library's foremost obligation to the other medical schools, and to the Medical Society and the medical community which had generously supported it, or which surrendered its books without strict guarantees of their full accessibility to the general profession. Since the BML for all practical purposes would be relinquishing alternative choices governing the use of its collections to an executive committee inevitably dominated by Harvard, it should insist that its own purposes be spelled out in an agreement and that their implementation be very clearly the joint responsibility of the partnership. Bradford foresaw some erosion of support for the BML if "it comes under the wing, or *appears to* come under the wing, of an institution as great as Harvard University," and advised that the profession should be assured by a stipulation in the agreement that the collections of each would be fully available to the community served by the other. He pressed the trustees to insist that space in the Countway Library be provided for the offices of *The New England Journal of Medicine*, for reading rooms and services for Fellows and members, and for the perpetuation or duplication of memorials.

With Dean Soutter in the dissent, the trustees directed President Sprague to appoint a representative committee to continue negotiations with Harvard. In March the Harvard Corporation approved the "Statement of Principles" in principle and Dean Berry's appointment of a committee for the Medical School.[16]

As the two institutions got down to the mechanics of collaboration, Dr. Soutter in his plainspoken manner carried his demurrer against Harvard domination into *The Boston Medical Quarterly*, of which he was editor and which was published by the Boston University School of Medicine and the Massachusetts Memorial Hospitals. Begging the editorial question, "The Boston Medical Library: Should Harvard Take It Over?"—the *BMQ* argued that regardless of the advantages of an alliance and the publicmindedness of Harvard, "if the Boston Medical Library comes under its control, it cannot help but be administered for the benefit of Harvard faculty and students first and of other doctors and other students second." Should BU and Tufts medical students and members of the Massachusetts Medical Society (most of them neither alumni nor faculty of Harvard) have to go to Harvard for access to the literature? And if the trustees have the legal right to transfer the Boston Medical Library to a university,

> can they in full conscience dispense with the new stacks, furnishings and equipment given by many donors to increase the usefulness of a library for all doctors and students? How happy will be the many current subscribers to the Arthur W. Allen Fund, which has done so much to improve the Library, if all of these improvements are scrapped, the building sold and the contents moved elsewhere for another purpose? The same might be asked of those who subscribed to the Frank H. Lahey Room. The Medical Library houses the *New England Journal of Medicine* and the *Journal of Bone and Joint Surgery.* Both are dependent for the excellence of their editing upon the proximity of the Library. Are they to be dumped into the street? Must they petition Harvard for housing? The Massachusetts Medical Society uses the hall in the top of the Library for meetings of its Council. Must it now turn to a university for a place to meet at a considerable distance from its headquarters?

The editorialist ruefully supposed that the trustees could legally enter into a merger. "This is a problem. The Officers of the Trustees are all members of the Harvard faculty and most of them strongly favor the transfer."[17]

Such devil's advocacy from one who was himself a Harvard Medical graduate, with Dr. Bradford's cautions and the remonstrance from Dr.

Charles C. Lund, president of the Medical Society, that its members and other patrons of the BML should be "thoroughly and happily taken care of," had their cumulative effect on the deliberations of the joint negotiators which opened on April 21.

The first trial balloon of compromise was released in an editorial in *The New England Journal of Medicine* on May 14, 1959, which stated that the BML had been assured it will remain a free public library, that the combined facilities will be open to all responsible persons and to the students of Boston University, Tufts or any other medical schools as "first-class users. . . there will be no second-class users in this respect." The editorial disclosed that Harvard had offered to house the BML and its two journal tenants in their own wing (a suggestion of separate but equal facilities which soon fell before the exigencies of cataloguing and traffic flow, and integration of the general collections triumphed). First the *Journal* proffered the carrot of collaboration (the Countway would be second only to the new National Medical Library at Bethesda), and then in eeyorish tones (Eeyore, the doleful donkey in *Winnie the Pooh,* was a favorite *bête brun* of the Editor's) rattled the stick of decline and possible fall:

> There is no indication that the Boston Medical Library under the present circumstances can continue very long to give adequate service as an independent enterprise; even with the current support of the Massachusetts Medical Society, so freely granted to it a dozen years ago in a carefully considered act of enlightened generosity, it cannot meet its obligations. . . The question how long this deficit financing can be maintained must be faced. . . The matter of how long the Boston Medical Library can continue to occupy a position of any importance as a rival rather than as a fully co-ordinated institution is not one to inspire optimism. Even with the unforunate duplication of effort and material that would be entailed, it might well survive this crisis as it has survived others, but its importance might become an antiquarian one rather than one of actively contributing to the progress of medicine.[18]

Substantive agreement was reached in June after a number of meetings and discussions. Richard Warren, chairman of the Harvard committee, outlined to Howard Sprague on the nineteenth the settled terms of collaboration and minor remaining points of difference, concluding: "We are all grateful to your group for having initially approached us with the proposal for union. It must be recognized, however, that since Harvard is putting up the larger amount of money and will be owning and maintaining the building, the Boston Medical Library will be called upon to sacrifice a fraction of its former independence and even a measure of control over its own destiny. My committee wishes me to assure the Boston Medical Library that Harvard will always be vitally interested in the preservation of its partner's identity and the perpetuation of its invaluable services to the medical public."[19] On June 24 the trustees accepted the Warren letter in principle.

At about the same time the mollified editor of *The Boston Medical Quarterly* applauded the progress of negotiations and expressed "great hope that a satisfactory arrangement can be reached whereby all physicians in New England and all students and faculty members will have access to an extraordinarily large and useful medical library housed in a new plant and well equipped to serve them."[20]

The way now was clear for the drafting of a "Letter of Agreement" which was endorsed by Harvard President Nathan M. Pusey and accepted by the Corporation on November 16. On the eighteenth it was approved tentatively by the Medical Library trustees. Minor changes acceptable to Harvard were written into it at the suggestion of Dean Soutter, who then withdrew his reservations, and on December 16 the trustees adopted it unanimously, subject to ratification by the Fellows of the Library. On Christmas Eve *The New England Journal* and Walter Phippen, the esteemed former president of Library and Medical Society, cheerfully blessed the impending event.[21] The Fellows of the Boston Medical Library at a special meeting on January 5, 1960 without dissent ratified the action of their trustees in uniting with the Fellows of Harvard College for the greater good of medicine.

The pact by which the Boston Medical Library entered what was intended to be an equal partnership with America's richest and most powerful university guaranteed its autonomy, its right to manage its own funds and its ownership of its collections and future accessions. Likewise, of course, Harvard. The Medical School agreed to build the Francis A. Countway Library of Medicine on its own land, to provide furnishings and equipment except for those brought along by its partner, to maintain and repair it, to reserve for the BML a trustees' room, an administrative office, a physicians' reading room and an area for books on the history of medicine (to be designated the Prince, Wadsworth, Fifield and Lahey rooms and Holmes and Ware halls), and to rent offices to *The New England Journal of Medicine* and *The Journal of Bone and Joint Surgery*, which agreed to supply the Countway, as they had their old landlord, with copies enough for a vigorous periodical exchange program. The headquarters of the Massachusetts Medical Society would remain at 22 The Fenway.

The collections of the two libraries, except for components owned under restrictions, were to be intershelved. The entire contents of the Countway were to be available without institutional distinction to medical students and faculties, research workers, physicians, dentists and others designated by the Librarian. The borrowing privilege would be restricted to Harvard Medical Center personnel, Fellows and members of the BML including medical student members from Boston University and Tufts, and cardholders of the Boston Public Library and other libraries with respect to books owned by those libraries and on deposit at the Countway. It was agreed that the Countway was to be the principal library for the Harvard Medical, Dental and Public Health schools, and a research and consultation facility for Boston University and Tufts, "whose own libraries it is thus intended to supplement but not to replace."

The first Librarian of the Countway would be Ralph Esterquest. His successors would be named by the Harvard Corporation on recommendation of the Faculty of Medicine and with the approval of the BML trustees. Charles Colby would be Associate Librarian for Boston Medical Library Services, responsible to the Librarian save respecting the affairs and books of the BML, for which he would be answerable to the trustees, who were to appoint his successors with the approval of the Harvard Corporation. The Countway would be administered by a Joint Library Committee comprised of three representatives of each partner and the Librarian *ex officio* as chairman with a tie-breaking vote only.[22] In the case of a tie on "party lines," however, the issue could be referred by either side for resolution to the Harvard Corporation and Boston Medical Library trustees, who in any event reserved the right of veto over any Joint Committee decision affecting their separate affairs. Members of the combined staff would be officers and employes of Harvard University.

First claim on the unrestricted funds of the Boston Medical Library (which would include the net proceeds of the presumed future sale of 8 The Fenway) would be an annual sum of up to $7000 for the operating expenses of the trustees. The balance, in order of priority, would be reserved to reimburse Harvard for eighty per cent of the Librarian's salary, then twenty per cent of the Associate Librarian's, then the BML's fair share of the joint operating expenses, which was established at twenty per cent of the annual total after deducting the compensation of the two librarians and the cost of the purchase, binding and repair of its own books. . . but not to exceed eighty per cent of the balance remaining after the librarians had been paid; the final claim on the unrestricted funds of the BML was the abovementioned book costs. Also spelled out in the agreement was the joint budget protocol.

Remote as were the chances of its invocation, there was even an escape clause allowing either party to terminate the agreement on two years' notice. . . with the understanding that the terminator "shall be responsible for the cost of removing the collections and any other property of BML from the new building to such other place in the City of Boston as may be designated by BML."

Dr. Earle M. Chapman was to represent the Boston Medical Library on the Building Committee.

While the final dimensions of this remarkable document were being hammered on the forge of destiny, the ever-resourceful Dean Berry and his associates were purchasing from the City of Boston the intersection of Shattuck Street and Huntington Avenue and the land adjoining the Longwood Quadrangle and the Peter Bent Brigham Hospital, and were in the convoluted process of having the end of the street wiped out as a public highway in order to make way for the largest academic medical library in the world.

On January 14, 1960, in Cambridge, President Pusey signed the covenant rejoining the path from which the first Boston Medical Library and Harvard's medical school had pursued their separate ways 134 years earlier. Five days later President Sprague signed for his Library, at Suva, in the Fiji Islands.

12

Union
1960 · 1974

The Boston Medical Library should remember that, without this fruitful union, it might well have ceased to exist. . . We have secured its corporate survival, but we are only one side of an arch, the keystone of which is the enthusiastic acceptance of the unity of the Countway Library.

Howard B. Sprague's farewell address[1]

Looking to the troth which would pledge the Boston Medical Library to dower the Harvard Medical School with its own houseful, Librarians Esterquest and Colby undertook several months in advance of the event to revamp Harvard's original plans for a bachelor manor into a more stately mansion (an old story for Holmes's chambered library) built for two.

The scale of the joint enterprise had been calibrated by March 1961, when a revised working edition of the Countway building program was circulated.[2] The usable space which in 1958 Esterquest had projected for the Medical School's needs, 92,650 square feet, emerged as 130,600 for the combined libraries. Bound book capacity was almost doubled from 389,500 to 750,000. An even thousand remained the live display of current journals, but as Dean Berry noted in a report to the Overseers' Visiting Committee,[3] the savings from eliminating 700 duplicated and expensive serials would cover the subscriptions to another thousand or more less costly ones now beyond the budgetary reach of either partner, not to mention other economies issuing from the merger in book purchases, employment, maintenance and so on. Journals and books ten years old and younger would be segregated in the new set-up and somewhat more easily available than their elders and ancestors, according to their topicality and popularity.

Since the open stack policy would prevail (they were open in Building A but never at 8 The Fenway), several miles of them would confront the unfamiliar reader with labyrinthine choices; everywhere within reach of the desperate at the Countway would be an Ariadnean thread, a red telephone network plugged into the library staff by which the lost would be redirected to the path to enlightenment. The square footage originally reserved for the School's archival and faculty collections was greatly enlarged to accommodate (it was hoped, a little nervously) the amorphous historical collections of the BML and of the medical societies deposited with it, and its only superficially excavated cellarful of rarities, curiosities, souvenirs and hand-me-downs of successions of compulsive collectors. In only one respect did the vision shrink in the rethinking: seats for readers were reduced from 740 to 650.

Indeed, the first plan retained so nearly intact the essentials of its shape and purpose, expanding merely in size to embrace the worldly goods of the aged bride, as to add credence to the suspicion that it was an outcome the planners had hoped for, if not banked on, from the outset.

As to design, the architect was instructed in the revised building program that his blueprints "must reflect the fundamental policy that the totality of the Countway Library serves without distinction both Harvard and non-Harvard readers," that they must take into account that many users of the BML were less sophisticated about scientific developments and less familiar with the literature than Harvard people, that workers in different disciplines used the literature differently, that the humanities would find the climate warmer in the Countway than in the Medical School, and that "those who design the building should remember that the emphasis is not on housing books but on housing readers using books. . . Ideally, the reader should be able, upon stepping through the front door, to see at once the several important services—reserve books, new periodicals, indexes, public catalogs, etc.—and to know where he wants to go."[4]

In May 1962 Hugh A. Stubbins and Associates of Cambridge had finished the general architectural plans and drawings. They incorporated some further refinements. The Countway was set on a course of enlarging and streamlining the BML's ongoing regional circulation service that Dean Berry saw as the base for making it the New England reservoir in a system canalled via other such at New York, Baltimore and Philadelphia with the greatest of all reserves, the National Library of Medicine at Bethesda.[5] Photocopying would replace lending of periodicals, and although contemporary application of computer technology to library service was regarded with some skepticism, provision was to be built in for taking advantage of advances in electronic communication and information retrieval.

The *core* theme of the Countway had emerged. "A basic principle of the design," in Esterquest's words, "is that movement of people—and attendant commotion—will take place around a central core. Journals and books will be found in a kind of ring area that surrounds this core. The reader, having selected his book, will find a comfortable chair or chair and table immediately at hand, not a long walk away in a conventional reading room. . . A feature of the design is repose—a sense of things being open rather than closed in and aesthetic qualities that please the eye and nourish the soul."[6]

Moreover, the limitations of the site itself imposed a vertical slant on the traditional horizontal conception of the library. It was a case of necessity and invention. Hugh Stubbins was struck that "a central open space running through floors seemed to fulfill the spirit of the program in expressing the openness and accessibility of the information to be stored in the building. . . Outwardly, it seemed important that this building—the heart of the School—be a strong addition to the group, and not overpowered by the Medical School's classical buildings; but it also seemed important to be on speaking terms with the other permanent buildings even though it was necessary to use another vocabulary to express the age in which the Library was to be built."[7] Actually, the west corner of the Countway crowded the Brigham, which didn't at the time come under the architect's definition of a "permanent" building, one supposes, since it was eventually to be torn down to make way for the Associated Hospitals complex which has since become snarled in neighborhood problems.

Working drawings for the monument to her brother were nearing completion when Sanda Countway died on March 31, 1963 at eighty-one. "I'm sure we can be forgiven," Esterquest said, "if we think of it as a memorial to her as well, and to her uncommon understanding and public spirit."[8] The chain reaction which Miss Countway's thoughtful munificence had set off—Harold Vanderbilt's launching of the endowment and then the Markle Foundation grant—had ignited the involvement of other national foundations in the implications of the Countway experiment for adjustment to the explosion of knowledge, if not for its containment. The Rockefeller Foundation gave $1,500,000, the Commonwealth Fund $600,000, the Susan P. Baker Trust $373,754, the Avalon Foundation $150,000, the James Foundation $100,000, the Ford Motor Company Fund $100,000, the James J. and M. Sears Minot Family Foundation $50,310, the Godfrey M. Hyams Trust $25,000, others in lesser amounts. . . and the eight million dollars which Dean Berry had declared *would* be raised, *was* raised.

On May 12, 1964 ("to contain my sense of exhilaration on this occasion is difficult," exulted the Dean) the cornerstone of the Francis A.

Countway Library of Medicine was laid, and a sealed box containing a few items of curiosity for bigger builders of the future to discover sealed therein. The ceremonies were presided over by President Pusey of Harvard and participated in by President Sprague of the Boston Medical Library, the deans of the *four* medical schools (the University of Massachusetts School of Medicine now existed in the person of Dean Soutter), the president of the Massachusetts Medical Society, the librarians, and Dr. Burwell, who traced the history of the medical libraries of Boston to the instant moment, which "makes the future brighter for all people interested in medicine and in scholarship; for teachers, for investigators, and for those who care for patients."[9]

Would that the contents of the Countway could have been catalogued as compatibly as they were integrated! When collaboration was a certainty in the fall of 1959, the two staffs began laying plans for coordinating their cataloguing so that on moving day they could promptly interfile and intershelve their recent collections and catalogues. They agreed not to reclassify or recatalogue the bulk of their old collections on the assumption that the use of these would decline over the years and serve chiefly the needs of scholars. After the libraries had amalgamated Howard Sprague referred to their "friendly, but somewhat aloof relationship, like two dusty drops of mercury upon a watch glass. But. . . if you clean the surface of such drops, make them shine, and give each a clearer vision of his neighbor, their surface tensions will subside and they will instantly flow together and become one, especially if you give them a slight jolt."[10] A charming fancy, but as Ann T. Curran, research assistant in the Countway recalled, rather more than a nudge was necessary to pool the periodicals:[11]

> The two libraries used different schemes for recording and shelving their serials. Harvard's serial record entered the *Journal of the American Medical Association* under "Journal;" the Boston Medical entered it under "American." Harvard alphabetized its records by significant words ignoring all articles, prepositions, and conjunctions; Boston Medical filed by every word. Harvard shelved its journals in open stacks, alphabetically by title; Boston Medical shelved its journals in closed stacks by shelf location number. About one-fifth of the serials in the Harvard Medical Library had been catalogued; the Boston Medical Library had only a holdings record. At Harvard, an ACME 5 x 8" visible file was used to check in current receipts; at Boston Medical, current issues were checked in on 3 x 5" cards.

There were, in fact, some 17,000 different serial titles in various sizes, shapes and handwriting, a Procrustean problem which was first assaulted by photocopying them all to fit cards of 5 x 8. Then followed the intricate and intense team project of bringing the disparities into alphabetized uniformity—the better part of a year's job in Holmes Hall—

and ultimately recording it all on punched cards for consumption by whatever machines feed on such alphabet soup.

Whether through the perversity of a sometimes kind fate, or through the contagion of success sometimes transmitted by no more than the distant prospect of a financial liaison with awesome Harvard, the fortunes of the Boston Medical Library seemed to swing upwards once its future had been taken care of in the Letter of Agreement to which its President, sojourning among the Fijis, had affixed his signature. That very year, sixty-one new members signed on. A marked shift in the pattern of use emerged. While attendance dropped from 16,875 in 1954 to about 12,000 in 1960, a circulation increase from 72,875 to nearly 125,000 would have been gratifying if it were not so shattering to the budget. In following the course of regional service which had been plotted for it in 1940, when it outfitted a traveling library as the back-up for a series of courses offered by the Committee on Postgraduate Instruction of the Massachusetts Medical Society, the Medical Library had extended its clientele to the farthest corners of New England, and at considerable cost.

Use increased, and so did the endowment, belying fears that the supposition that the BML had a sugar daddy in Harvard would shut off support from its old constituency. The Library received the largest strictly professional bequest in its history, $100,000 for periodicals, from Dr. Beth Vincent, who died on July 11, 1962. From Fort Dodge, Iowa, where he was born in 1876, Vincent had migrated east, graduated from Harvard College and the Medical School in 1902, trained at the MGH and remained on its surgical staff until his retirement in 1935 when he was succeeded by Arthur Allen as chief of the East Surgical Service. He was an early worker in hematology with Roger I. Lee and Paul D. White, and with them developed the blood coagulation time assay variously known as the Lee-White method and Lee-Vincent test which made feasible his invention of the Vincent direct transfusion tube in 1913. His later interest in pediatric surgery led to his special assignment in 1930 as the MGH's first surgeon to children. Dr. Vincent had been a member of the BML for more than half a century.

That same year of 1962 Mrs. Margaret Farlow Castle followed a generous parental example and gave the Library $10,000 in memory of her father. The Vincent and Castle gifts led in raising the portfolio to a market value in 1963 of approximately $1,250,000, and earnings to $36,000. The Medical Library's gross income now verged on the $100,000 which George Berry in 1960 had anticipated *after* investment of the net proceeds from the sale of its real estate in order to justify his projected initial Countway budget of $436,000.[12] Yet the year at Number 8 ended $16,000 in the hole, with the move to the Countway less than twenty-four months away. Neither the sale of the Fenway property nor the Bell bequest (Mrs. Bell was very much alive) had materialized.

Nearly a year before the Letter of Agreement was signed, the New England Historic Genealogical Society had indicated its interest in buying 8 The Fenway in the face of the state's intended eminent domain seizure of its headquarters and library on Beacon Hill.[13] Negotiations proceeded so satisfactorily that on May 16, 1962 the BML trustees voted to accept an offer of $300,000. Nine months later the deal was off. Under pressure from the state, the Society needed new quarters by September of 1964, and the Countway would not be ready for occupancy until the spring after. The Society withdrew its offer in favor of a location on Newbury Street. As luck would have it, a few doors down from the Library the Boston Conservatory of Music was looking for room to expand. Talks moved along rapidly, and on January 15, 1964 the trustees agreed to sell to the Conservatory for the same price, $300,000. (The actual sale did not occur until after the move to the Countway, in July 1965, and the Library vacated its old home on September 2.)

On June 14, 1965 the Boston Medical Library closed its doors as an independent society. For two days it disgorged its contents to merge with those of the Harvard Medical Library in a single stream that trickled, poured and flooded into the empty stacks, the miles of them, in the Francis A. Countway Library of Medicine. On June 16 the Countway opened to readers.

When that first Boston Medical Library invited the patronage of its members in the waning days of 1805, it displayed forty-two volumes in John Fleet's drawing room. At the end of 1875, Chadwick's revival of it in the already overcrowded confines of Hamilton Place boasted 1849 books, 2639 bound volumes of journals, 3000 pamphlets and 120 periodicals subscribed to. Eighty-eight years later, after thirty-five tons of literature had been weeded out and shipped off for recycling in preparation for the move, there remained on the last day of 1964 for trucking over to the Countway 97,267 monographs (mostly books), 129,665 volumes of periodicals and 7121 volumes of dissertations, which together with miscellaneous categories made a total of 245,643 volumes. They occupied, by the estimate of Librarian Colby, about four running miles of shelves. For its part, the Harvard Medical Library contributed 69,691 monographs, 79,849 serials and 5238 volumes of dissertations, adding up with its odd books to 166,514.

Thus the Countway offered the disciminating reader 412,157 hopefully catalogued volumes of knowledge to choose from, or ten thousand times the amount (numerically, anyway) that was placed at the disposal of the Boston profession from the Milk Street quarters of Dr. Fleet on that distant day of 1805. It took six months following the move for a crew under the direction of Mrs. Charles Colby to interfile the 315,000 catalogue cards of the two libraries. The move cost the BML $98,210, the Medical School $60,996.

Richard J. Wolfe, a University of Pittsburgh graduate and bibliographic scholar specializing in early printing, came to the Countway as Rare Books Librarian from the Lilly Library of Indiana University, and he attacked the unbelievable lode that had been excavated from the Fenway and avalanched into his department with the excitement of a first-strike Klondike prospector.

There was, for instance, that vexatious but highly prized library on pharmacology and toxicology of Professor Kobert which Director Ballard had picked up as a bargain in Rohrbach. . . the one they had such trouble getting out after the Armistice, and which so embarrassed Dr. Farlow in 1927 when he had to admit to the members that the fine Kobert collection "remains untouched in its boxes in the basement, I am sorry to say." And in the basement is where Wolfe and Colby found it, still crated, thirty-eight years later.

And then there were the three letters from Edward Jenner to Benjamin Waterhouse which were unearthed during the move and rejoined with a collection of Waterhouse material from which they had been inexplicably separated and which had come to the Rare Books Department by its own route from the Medical School, where it had been on deposit. When the author happened to ask Mr. Wolfe if he could shed any light on a certain entry in the trustees' minutes, the mystery was reduced to another case of absentmindedness at 8 The Fenway.

Henry Viets had advised the trustees on December 15, 1941 (as their minutes recorded) that Reginald Fitz of the Medical School's committee on library had written him of the finding of a note in the back of a scrapbook of Waterhouse material stating that three or four letters from Jenner had been loaned to the Boston Medical Library on January 23, 1903. The scrapbook included correspondence from Presidents Jefferson, Madison and John Quincy Adams and had been deposited with the Harvard Medical Library by Mrs. W. R. Thayer of Cambridge. Naturally, Dr. Fitz would appreciate the return of the Jenner letters after the passage of thirty-eight years. Dr. Viets told the trustees that he and Mr. Ballard had searched high and low, with no success whatever; probably the letters had been borrowed for a meeting and no doubt long since given back and somehow mislaid at the Medical School. Satisfied, the board instructed him to notify Fitz that "there is no evidence or record" that the Jenner-Waterhouse correspondence is at the Boston Medical Library.

When such stars crossed, the revelation of twenty-one incunabula misplaced or forgotten altogether stretched credulity no thinner. One actually found its loser. It was a first edition of the *Margarita poetica* by Albrecht von Eyb, published in Nuremberg by Johann Sensenschmidt on December 2, 1472. Upon its discovery and return to the light of day, this large and brilliantly illustrated treasure caught the eye of Curator Viets. Something about it was vaguely familiar, and he left it at that because he was engaged in sorting through the papers he planned to bring over to the Countway. Among them he shortly came upon his diary of a trip to Europe in the summer of 1932 with Harvey Cushing and Arnold Klebs, the incunabulist. At Munich, on the evening of September 6, the bibliophiles called on the booksellers Taeuber and Weil:

> The genial Taeuber and the scholarly Dr. Weil had provided a rare feast for their guests. They had recently acquired some books from the famous Benedictine Abbey at Ottobeuern, formerly the property of Ulrich von Ellenbog, a fifteenth-century physician and collector, who died in 1499. A score or more of the volumes were lined upon a table for inspection. When Cushing sat down before them, with Taeuber and Weil discretely in the background, the Curator fortunately took a photograph with his Leica of the group completely absorbed in their respective tasks. There, in the very center of the row, was the bulky incunable, the *Margarita poetica* of von Eyb, unmistakable in size and shape. Since Cushing did not buy it, the book was promptly ordered by the Curator for the Boston Medical Library.
>
> Thus, through a timely snapshot and the penchant of the Curator for keeping an illustrated diary, the mystery of the acquisiton of the volume was at last resolved. When it reached the Library and why the book was never accessioned is another matter.
>
> Munich in 1932 was not a restful place for learned booksellers of Jewish extraction. Hitler came into full power the next year, and Dr. Weil escaped to London, where he carried on his profession in an admirable manner until his death early in 1965. What happened to the book during the unstable period of the Nazi regime and how it got to Boston or when it arrived is not known. But the volume, so briefly seen but fully identified in 1932, now rests safely on the Library shelves.[14]

One hypothesis to account for at least some of these amnesic lapses in the special collections of the Boston Medical Library is couched in archeological terms by Harold Bloomquist, who was the Assistant Librarian of the Harvard Medical Library in the pretransfenway period: desiring to project the most generous possible dimensions for their rare books department, the planners had made sample "borings" into what they supposed was the deepest interior of the cellars and coal bins of 8 The Fenway. But on moving day to their dismay, when the diggers were sent in, the appalling discovery was made that the test borers had never so much as penetrated the crust of the core of the hoard and had consequently underestimated the enormity of it by half, with the result that the Rare Books Department had to be ruptured into proximal space and doubled in size. Ralph Esterquest put the best face on it:

> Predecessor librarians in both libraries, but particularly in the Boston Medical Library, gathered on their shelves—and, I may add, in their closets, attics, and cellars—enormous numbers of books and, included among them, a great many treasures. Thousands of these books are reasonably well catalogued, but many more thousands are unlisted and unrecorded. In the months, and perhaps years ahead, we will have the pleasure of discovery as we work our way through what we playfully call our "deferred maintenance."[15]

One sentimental favorite of several generations of Boston medicine was missing from the van on the day of the move, not because it had been misplaced, but because it had been loaned to the MGH, which was loath to give it back. This was a huge painting of John Collins Warren operating on Gilbert Abbott in the first public demonstration of ether anesthesia under the Bulfinch Dome on October 16, 1846, all of eight feet by ten. It had been presented to the Library in 1903 by the artist, Robert Hinckley of Washington. For many years it half-covered the wall behind the speaker's dais in Ware Hall, where a spotlight was fixed on the white figure of the young patient. In 1946 this cloud of canvas was cleaned at Dr. David Cheever's expense and loaned to the hospital for the Ether Centennial, returned (after some dragging of feet) and loaned again in 1963. In 1974 the "Ether Painting" was back in the neutral hands of the restorer, while the issue of whose wall it should honor was provoking the division of some passionate institutional loyalties.

George Packer Berry would be relaying the guidance of the Harvard Medical School to Dr. Robert H. Ebert on June 30, 1965, and so it was no less than fitting that his *summum opus* should be dedicated on May 26 and 27 during the final Alumni Week of his singular deanship. A tent was pitched over the plaza (and the stacks without end of medical literature underneath it) for a thousand guests. Men of note came to delve on the first day into "The Significance of Medical History" and on the second into "The Scientific Information Problem" and "Challenge of the New Technology," all culminating on the afternoon of the twenty-seventh with the dedicatory address by the poet and former Librarian of Congress, Archibald MacLeish, and the formal dedication by President Pusey.[16]

Harvard's view of the sublimation of the suit that several generations of its servants had pursued sporadically (though nonetheless never unremittingly for long) was expressed in magnanimous yet firm tones by him who in the end had won the hand. Declared Dean Berry:

> After more than 150 years of marriage and divorce, of reunion and separation—of peaceful coexistence in latter years—we of the Harvard Medical School and our colleagues at the Boston Medical Library have engaged for nearly a decade in careful planning and negotiation, guided by the conviction that through union we could better meet the challenges of postwar medicine. . .
>
> In former years, when medical education and medical knowledge were growing at a pace less rapid than we know today, a library of 20,000 or 30,000 volumes could reasonably well meet the requirements of a medical school or medical society. It was not—in those more leisurely times—inappropriate for a community to support two medical libraries: one for the medical school; the other for medical practitioners. This dual arrangement was not only possible, it mirrored the separate ways of life in academic cloisters and the market place. In the present era of unprecedented growth and of the ever-closer involvement of university medicine in society, such a pattern is no longer wise or practical. The problem is in part one of quantity—being able to absorb and pay for the tremendous outpouring of medical literature; in part one of quality—being able to mobilize pertinent information from widely scattered sources; and in part one of speed—being able to do so rapidly and effectively. It is important that the practitioner as well as the academician, whether teacher or student, have ready access to the collections and services of a university medical library, lest he become isolated from the moving front of discovery.
>
> The solution lies in recognizing the interdependence and facilitating the cooperation by which medical libraries can extend their reach. This goal has been superbly met in the new Countway. Its combined collections will be made freely available to the entire medical community: to the students and faculties of all the medical schools and their teaching hospitals in Massachusetts, and to physicians and hospitals throughout New England. Thus, the Countway will function for a large geographic area as a regional reservoir library. In partnership with the National Library of Medicine and with projected regional libraries in other large medical centers, the Countway will eventually be part of a nationwide network.[17]

To Archibald MacLeish, the humanist, if success should crown this hitherto untried effort to transcend the traditional custodial function of the library by carrying scientific information straight to the practitioner, "it will have connected the republic of common knowledge with parts at least of that revolutionary frontier which so often seems to turn its back, like all frontiers, on the peopled lands behind it."[18]

The notion that the Countway might itself create a frontier in medical communication by extending routes between his moving front of discovery and the poet's republic of common knowledge (and in the process interest a foundation or two in providing the remaining three million dollars he needed) had been conveyed to the Visiting Committee by Dean Berry as far back as 1960.[19] The webbing upon which the new design was woven was the existing regional service furnished its members for years by the Boston Medical Library, albeit starved the while for funds. To build on this commitment, the Extra-Mural Services Office was set up in the Countway, at first on a short budget. Then in 1965 Congress passed the Medical Library Assistance Act, and regional service planning was at once a viable activity. A year later the library became a New England regional search center (though not thoroughly functioning until 1967) for MEDLARS, the Medical Literature Analysis and Retrieval System, a computerized program of the National Library of Medicine built around Dr. Billings's *Index Medicus*, to make quickly available to the requester a large part of the world bibliography of biomedical literature, as well as selected subject bibliographies of ineffable sophistication.

In June 1967 the Countway was designated the New England Regional Medical Library for the National Library of Medicine, the first of eleven in the nation, so chosen on account of the service the BML was already providing in the area, mainly through the professional memberships. The new regional service (NERMLS) got going in October as an expansion of the Extra-Mural Services Office; NERMLS was linked with MEDLARS for the benefit of institutions and individuals beyond a half a mile of the Countway lacking ready access to a medical library.

Another year, and in August 1968 the Countway was tied in to another galaxy of computerized communication as one of nine participating libraries in the System for Medical and Biological Sciences Information Searching (SYMBIOSIS) which enabled the information-seeker actually to pose his questions to a keyboard in English (if he remembered any at this point) instead of code. SYMBIOSIS was a creature of the Biomedical Communications Network (BCN) of the component medical centers of SUNY (the State University of New York). News of this latest acronymic triumph was too much for BML Secretary Chapman, who felt constrained to comment mournfully in the minutes of October that "for the first time, the Sunday-supplement kind of futuristic picture of a physician pushing a button and a computer spewing out information for him is a partial reality."

Some cold comfort for the unreconstructably old-fashioned was squeezed from the fate of Ralph Esterquest's experiment in providing all comers to the Countway with free and unlimited photocopying service as the alternative to lending periodicals:

> "You'll be sorry!" said the sideline observers. We had excellent people on the desk dealing with the hungry, copy-mad readers. Among other things, we observed that modern copy techniques have created a new phenomenon that we have called "copying in lieu of reading."

> Suffice it to say, we kept busy, and the copy traffic steadily increased as the summer wore on. When August [1965] statistics were in, they told us that the service—at the *August* level—would cost, on an annual basis, approximately $110,000. So, we threw in the sponge, and the Wednesday after Labor Day was the last free copy day in the Countway. Indeed, we spent another week cleaning up Wednesday's accumulation. Our non-lending policy—remember—was aimed at keeping periodicals in the Library and in their proper places on the shelves. They stayed in the Library all right, but most of them were downstairs in the Copy Service room.[20]

After nine years as President of the Boston Medical Library, during which he had devoted himself—in spite of, or possibly because of, his deep conservatism—to pulling and coaxing the fellowship from the pleasant and musty vagaries of the Victorian age to face the bewildering efficiencies of the electronic, Howard B. Sprague retired at the annual meeting on April 17, 1967 with a typical parting shaft:

> Now we confront the faceless computer, gleaming and flashing; not covered with the dust of antiquity and personal recondite exploration, as was Jim Ballard. Yet it seems to be little known that the principle of the punch card and computer, from which has grown the mammoth IBM Company, was the invention of a medical librarian, Dr. John Shaw Billings, who started the system in 1880. He foresaw the problem of storage and retrieval, and, no doubt, the necessary impersonality of the machine almost ninety years ago.
>
> Our librarians are inheritors of his vision and vibrantly aware of the bibliographical giant that has expanded out of the constant rubbing of the lamp of knowledge. I am sure they would like the medical scientist to stop rubbing the lamp for a while to let them catch up.[21]

His successor was Joseph Garland, who also had concluded to retire, after twenty years as Editor of *The New England Journal of Medicine* the next month, and not wishing to slip from the traces all at once, had consented as well to re-assume the direction of the *Harvard Medical Alumni Bulletin,* of which he had been the first editor in 1927. At seventy-four, Garland was the oldest president in the history of the Boston Medical Library, and long active in its affairs. Son and grandson of general practitioners in the ancient fishing port of Gloucester, he had graduated from Harvard College in 1915 and the Medical School in 1919, trained at the MGH and practised pediatrics for a quarter of a century before taking over the *Journal*, with everything that this second career evoked for him of his earliest love, literature and writing. Bentley P. Colcock, a surgeon at the Lahey Clinic, was elected vice president, and George T. Bottomley treasurer.

The Garland administration spanned a hiatus of some uncertainty. The partnership with Harvard had come off smoothly enough. The collections had been intershelved and the catalogues interfiled, or were somewhere in comfortable contiguity, and the staffs were integrated in the employ of the University. The balance of power in the Countway as a unified library, however, and its future, were weighted subtly but unmistakably toward the Medical School. The Letter of Agreement guaranteed the institutional integrity of the Boston Medical Library, but it did not assure it of its continuing identity or set it upon a course of its own as the minority partner which sacrificed that "fraction of its former independence and even a measure of control over its own destiny" given notice of by Richard Warren. As President Garland saw it:

> There seemed, to the excessively cautious, some risk that eventually a benevolent paternalism might result in the absorption of the smaller and less opulent institution by the larger one, through a sort of benign phagocytosis.[22]

Fortunately, as a start in charting a new course, or hewing to an old one, a healthy independent income can spread the options, as it frequently does within a marriage, although there was little in the Countway budget to hold out much hope that two libraries could really live as cheaply as one.

After the first year of combined operation, Librarians Esterquest and Colby produced an accounting which revealed that the cost to the Countway of the average over-the-desk loan to a BML member was fifty-three cents, of a postal loan $1.30, of an interlibrary loan $4.35, and of a mere consultation of the collections, twenty-nine cents. They thought the dues ought to be increased. In October 1966 the trustees approved the first such rise since 1927, when the assessment for Fellows had gone from twelve to fifteen dollars; henceforth, all classes except medical students would pay twenty-five dollars.[23] The result was a predictable drop in responses to membership invitations to incoming fellows of the Massachusetts Medical Society. In October of the next year the trustees were seriously worried about membership maintenance, a problem of erosion which some were afraid would be aggravated by a slow loss of professional fellowships, now that the regional service the institutional and commercial members had been supporting was coming under the federal funding of the New England Regional Medical Library Service of the Countway. Was the Boston Medical Library having identity troubles already? The trustees wondered.

Ralph T. Esterquest, Dean Berry's foreign minister who had pieced together the pattern of partnership with such diplomacy and flair, died suddenly on August 10, 1968 at the age of only fifty-six. Gazing down from a high nearby building at his almost completed work one spring evening in 1965 with his assistant, Esterquest had sized up softly but emphatically his finest accomplishment: "That's one hell of a library."[24]

The assistant, Harold Bloomquist, succeeded him. He was a graduate of Albion College in 1950 and the Columbia School of Library Service in 1954 and had been brought by his predecessor to the Harvard Medical Library in 1958 as his assistant librarian for resources and acquisitions.

Since before the union Harvard had been after the Boston Medical Library to hand over its endowment for management, a proposition which had provoked inconclusive debate. Three months after Ralph Esterquest's death, Henry C. Meadow, Associate Dean for Financial Affairs at the Medical School, was invited to present the case for the affirmative before the trustees. The endowment in 1969 was inching up toward a million and a half and was expected to produce $60,000. Meadow proposed that the board relieve itself of its investment cares and turn this portfolio over to the University to manage as a trust. Admittedly, it probably would earn no more, but book values would be raised thereby to realistic levels; the funds would be further diversified, and there was a chance that the management fee could be reduced. Under some amiable questioning, the Associate Dean conceded that the BML would also thereby lose control of its money and likely never get it back. As an alternative Meadow suggested that Harvard could intermingle the BML's holdings with its own, in which case they could be reassembled and returned on demand. The board sat on Harvard's offer for a month, and in December finally tabled it.

Mrs. Bettye Bell died in July 1968. Throughout 1969 and into the next year the installments of her husband's bequest poured in by the hundreds of thousands. When the last check had been deposited in November of 1970, and the whole was added up, the Library's million and a half of capital funds, scrimped and saved over ninety-five years of Boston frugality, was blanketed not by $400,000 hoped for in 1955 after the demise of Dennistoun Bell, but under $1,078,604.92 derived from a few productive years in the war against indigestion, cholera morbus and vertigo.

This great legacy rather stiffened the grip of the smaller partner. And further did the decision of Tufts University to obtain for its 280 medical students the borrowing privilege in the Countway under the Letter of Agreement, by way of their membership in the BML at five dollars each. Boston University did not do likewise, as the medical school was expanding its own library, but in 1971 Dean Soutter's University of Massachusetts Medical School, which had opened for the fall term of 1970 in Worcester, also took out student memberships. And then came a truly exhilarating dose of financial adrenalin when, with admirable appreciation of the Countway's importance to the profession in Massachusetts, the Fellows of the Medical Society at their annual meeting in 1971 voted to double their BML dues to ten dollars. This single commitment to recurring support was the equivalent of the earnings from three quarters of a million dollars in endowment.

When Joseph Garland after four years passed the presidency in 1971 to Bentley Colcock (Charles Bradford was elected vice president, and Grant Rodkey replaced Earle Chapman as secretary), the Boston Medical Library had weathered the first stage of transition and improved its financial position up to a point where that year it was in a position to contribute $120,000 to the Countway budget, and still more the next, $152,000.

On the other hand, the roster of regulars had been shrinking too steadily since the opening of the combined library and that necessary dues increase, and the trustees felt no little concern for the future as they looked around them at their aging colleagues. The time must come when time would take its toll of those senior supporters who kept up their dues out of sentiment for old times, and if some new interests attracting new generations of members did not replace the fading memories of 8 The Fenway and anecdotes of the halcyon days of Jim Ballard, the BML as an organic entity was headed for oblivion.

As early as 1957, when the apparition of a new Harvard Medical Library first shimmered on their horizon, the trustees wondered with a certain apprehension what measures should be taken to protect and keep together their enormous cache of rare and historical literature. As the partnership took shape, this possessive concern was fortunately shared with the Medical School's for its great archives and translated by the Agreement into the more encompassing History of Medicine floor which housed not only these combined special collections but the household gods which literally and symbolically each library, though predominantly the BML, carried upon its back to the new conjugal hearthside.

Here at the east end of the fifth floor was the Rare Books Department (overflowing into the fourth and sixth before the last of the underestimated mountain had been moved from The Fenway), its offices (the Fifield and Prince rooms) and reading room (Holmes Hall); the Lahey Room for physicians to relax and read in; the Allen Room for the trustees; the Ware Room for small meetings; the James Jackson Minot Room of the Medical School for larger gatherings; and the auditorium for the largest.[25]

Around the walls of the corridor which squared the central core, and in the memorial rooms, were hung the portraits of those generations of gentlemen of the old school of medicine in Boston which had smiled and stared down upon more generations of teacher and taught in the book-crowded quarters of Boylston Place, The Fenway, Mason, North Grove, Boylston and Shattuck streets. . . chaired, by silent acquiescence, by the Autocrat beaming forth in that likeness which he truly believed had caught him truest. Here on this floor was committed the past of the Boston profession which deserved to survive and an inheritance of medical learning and lore which surely has few if any equals in the world.

Up here was the soul, the spirit, the real identity, after it had vacated its own peculiar house and intershelved all its carefully bookplated general collections with its partner's, of the old Boston Medical Library. Or was it only the brittle contents of a fugitive cachet from some cracked and quaint saddlebag of a lost era, enshrining for sentiment's sake the rejected and the useless, as worn out as Dr. Holmes's rocking chair?

The most positive response to this challenge of the past took form in the founding of "The Countway Library Associates; Friends of the Rare Books Collection" in the autumn of 1966 with the idea in mind of stimulating wider interest in the history of medicine, supporting the Rare Books Department specifically and adding to the collections. The founding president was Lloyd E. Hawes, Boston radiologist and Honorary Curator of the Historical Collection in Radiology. David P. Boyd was vice president, and Rare Books Librarian Richard Wolfe secretary-treasurer.

The sage of the Associates at seventy-six was Henry Viets, actively occupied as Consultant to the History of Medicine Program of the Countway since 1965, when the merger had relieved him of his pleasant duties as Curator of the BML. Dr. Viets enjoyed the group the more for its assumption of the fallen mantle of the BML's old Boston Medical History Club, that cultural amphitheatre in which he had scrubbed so happily for Harvey Cushing forty years earlier. The last of the dynasty of strong individualists so uniquely identified with the Boston Medical Library, he weathered the transition good-humoredly, on hand as always with wise counsel and encouragement. Practitioner, scientist, historian, bibliophile, and above all, literate scholar, Henry Rouse Viets died on July 5, 1969 in his eightieth year. In his memory a rare books and manuscripts purchasing fund was established in the Countway.

Nature's abhorrence of an empty space and the New Englander's of throwing anything away, and the mere passage of time, assured an ever normal fallout of historical drift on the Rare Books Department which compounded the stratification and rendered the core which had already repelled the borers ever less accessible. Many of the accessions were outstanding, such as William Dameshek's collection of works on hematology received after his death in 1970 and the private library of Howard Sprague, who died the same year on November 4. Acquisitions by ones and twos presented no problem; it was the extensive accessions which had to be accepted en masse and stashed away for culling on some indefinite future day when and if the staff, which at the moment was bent on the uncrating of the Kobert collection or sifting through the rediscovered letters of Oliver Wendell Holmes, could get to it. Some material was accepted into the special collections to save it from the dump, such as early hospital records, or from dispersal, as the original volumes in the Treadwell Library of the Massachusetts General Hospital. Occasionally an attempt could be made to catalogue an important accession before it was snowed under. In the fall of 1971 the manuscript records of the Massachusetts Medical Society from its founding in 1781 to about 1900 were released from solitary confinement in the vault at 22 The Fenway to the custody of its former landlord. To finance the cataloguing of this mass of rich material, which included at least 4000 random pieces of correspondence, the trustees of the BML in March 1972 set up the Walter L. Burrage, M.D. Fund in memory of the long-time secretary of the Library and secretary-historian of the Society.

About half of the entire holdings of the Boston Medical Library brought to the Countway constituted the major part of the history of medicine collections. Their extent can only be speculated, but it must be well in excess of 100,000 rare books and pamphlets, prints, portraits, photographs, busts and medals; more thousands of medical curiosities, instruments and memorabilia enough to build a museum around; uncounted, uncatalogued, unknown manuscript pieces mounting probably into the millions; and an entire library, as well, of secondary sources on medical history.

The centennial was around the corner, and thoughts turned to Dr. Holmes, a useful figure on any occasion. Early in 1973 the trustees approved the founding of the Oliver Wendell Holmes Society by Charles Bradford and Grant Rodkey, to explore the role of the medical profession in contemporary society, an always fretting relationship which the founding president frequently pondered himself. In another respect as germane to the impending hundredth anniversary were Holmes's thoughts on the uses, if any, of antiquated medical books, shared with the members during the dedication of that remarkable hall at the rear of 19 Boylston Place on December 3, 1878:

Men were not all cowards before Agamemnon or all fools before the days of Virchow and Billroth. And apart from any practical use to be derived from the older medical authors, is there not a true pleasure in reading the accounts of great discoverers in their own words? I do not pretend to hoist up the Bibliotheca Anatomica of Mangetus and spread it on my table every day. I do not get out my great Albinus before every lecture on the muscles, nor disturb the majestic repose of Vesalius every time I speak of the bones he has so admirably described and figured. But it does please me to read the first description of parts to which the names of their discoverers or those who have first described them have become so joined that not even modern science can part them; to listen to the talk of my old volume as Willis described his circle and Fallopius his aqueduct and Varolius his bridge and Eustachius his tube and Monro his foramen—all so well known to us in the human body; it does please me to know the very words in which Winslow described the opening which bears his name, and Glissen his capsule and De Graaf his vesicle; I an not content until I know in what language Harvey announced his discovery of the circulation, and how Spigelius made the liver his perpetual memorial, and Malpighi found a monument more enduring than brass in the corpuscles of the spleen and the kidney.[26]

The Oliver Wendell Holmes Endowment of the Boston Medical Library for the support of the Rare Books Department was organized in the spring of 1973, with a goal of $3,500,000 by the centennial year of 1975, together with an additional $350,000 to equip the entire Countway with a fire-suppression system. Richard Warren was appointed the general chairman, with a large steering committee under Chairman Mark D. Altschule, Professor of Medicine at Harvard and Honorary Curator of Prints and Photographic Collections in the Countway, and Vice Chairman Charles H. Bradford. In October Lloyd E. Hawes succeeded Bentley P. Colcock as President of the Boston Medical Library, with George W. B. Starkey vice president and George E. Gifford, Jr., secretary.

The endowment campaign had not been long under way when former President Garland died on August 4, 1973 at eighty. The trustees that autumn established the Joseph Garland Memorial Fund within the Holmes Endowment, with Dr. Jean A. Curran as chairman, for the support of the contemplated Joseph Garland Librarian for Special Collections, described as "the keystone position in the future of the Boston Medical Library. . . combining philosophical reflection with practical activity. As such it seems a fitting tribute to Dr. Garland's life and interests."[27]

* * * *

Dr. Holmes was never backward with his advice, and in his enjoyable role (in spite of his protestations) as the figurehead of the Boston Medical

Library he could not refrain from offering another solid piece of it to his former anatomy students and a few others assembled in Boylston Place that December dedication day of 1878:

It is not necessary to maintain the direct practical utility of all kinds of learning. Our shelves contain many books which only a certain class of medical scholars will be likely to consult. There is a dead medical literature, and there is a live one. The dead is not all ancient, the live is not all modern. There is none, modern or ancient, which, if it has no living value for the student, will not teach him something by its autopsy. But it is with the live literature of his profession that the medical practitioner is first of all concerned.

Notes Index

Notes

1. A DIMINUTIVE COMMENCEMENT

1. The portrait of Nicholas Boylston in the Countway is an embellished copy by Copley of his original.

2. Oliver Wendell Holmes, *Additional Memoranda* to "Medicine in Boston" by Samuel A. Green, in: Justin Winsor, *The Memorial History of Boston* (Boston, 1881), IV, 565.

3. *Ibid*, 566.

4. James Thacher, *American Medical Biography* (Boston, 1828), I, 304. Howard's portrait by Gilbert Stuart hangs in the Countway.

5. Holmes's *Memoranda,* 563.

6. It is of passing interest that John Collins Warren, Howard and Fleet shared another enthusiasm, that of their mentor, John Warren, for the Massachusetts Humane Society which he had founded with Waterhouse (when they were on speaking terms) and others and presided over from 1799 until 1813, two years before his death. Besides its famous concern for the shipwrecked, the Humane Society interested itself in the mystery of animation and the challenge of resuscitation. Howard delivered the annual discourse on the subject in 1804, and Fleet in 1797, proposing that "to me it appears, that there is but one principle, or spirit of animation—that muscular fibres contain a larger proportion than the nerves, and this is the vis plastica, or vis conservatrix naturae, for the purpose of preserving and propagating the several species of animated nature. Some animals possess this property to such a degree, as to be able to renew a part or whole of their bodies, as the crab, snail and polipe, and others regard but little the loss of their head, as the tortoise and toad."

Contemporary attempts at restoration of life employed "fumigators" to blow tobacco smoke up the bowels of the doubly unfortunate victim. In preparing his *The Humane Society of the Commonwealth of Massachusetts* (Cambridge, 1918), 26-27, Mark A. DeWolfe Howe inquired of several physician acquaintances whether there was any physiological rationale to this approach. "The most encouraging reply that has been received," he related, "was the counter-query: 'Wouldn't it make you sit up?' "

7. Winsor's *Memorial History*, IV, 282.

8. A *second* Second Social Library put in a phantom appearance in 1805, to fade from the record after a dozen years, leaving behind only a catalogue of 1808 that reveals its character as a general library and its claim to have been founded in January of 1805 and incorporated in 1806; a second edition carried a supplement listing books added between 1809 and 1811. Charles K. Bolton, Librarian of the Athenaeum, concluded that the Boston Medical Library was indeed the

Second Social, in his study, "Social Libraries in Boston," *Publications of the Colonial Society of Massachusetts* XII (1909), 332-338.

9. John W. Farlow, *The History of the Boston Medical Library* (Boston, 1918), 23.

10. John C. Warren, John G. Coffin and Asa Bullard were the trustees in 1808. Warren had succeeded Jackson. Dartmouth graduate Bullard and Coffin were two of the four to receive the first degrees of doctor of medicine awarded by Harvard in 1811.

11. Unless the Medical School was in error, the eleven hundred volumes given by Boylston in 1800 had shrunk unaccountably in ten years. Its second circular from Boston in 1811 stated that the Boylston collection "contains about seven hundred volumes selected with great care, relating to all the branches of medical sciences."

12. Farlow's *History*, 17.

13. The Boston Society for Medical Improvement was vigorously resuscitated by another generation of optimists in 1828, accompanied by the consumption of much tobacco smoke, no doubt.

14. Samuel Adams Drake, *Old Landmarks and Historic Personages of Boston* (Boston, 1872), 317.

15. Holmes's *Memoranda*, 564.

16. Drake's *Old Landmarks*, 317.

17. The BML catalogue for 1823 lists 1383 volumes. It's unlikely that these increased half again in three years. Still, libraries always discover hidden treasures at moving time.

18. Josiah Quincy, *The History of the Boston Athenaeum* (Cambridge, 1851).

2. HIBERNATION

1. Meeting of the Boston Society for Medical Improvement. *Boston Medical and Surgical Journal* CXLIV:11 (March 14, 1901), 259.

2. *Ibid*, 247.

3. Vincent Y. Boyditch, *Life and Correspondence of Henry Ingersoll Bowditch* (Boston, 1902), I, 49. Fifty-nine years later, in a letter in the *BMSJ* on August 25, 1892, Holmes referred to the *fight*, with the comment: "He was right and I was wrong."

4. John Ware, forty, was a late bloomer in medicine, having tried dentistry, schoolteaching and tutoring, the lecture circuit, the writing of fiction and poetry, and medical and non-medical editing, including a year with Walter Channing putting out the *BMSJ* in 1828, before James Jackson made a professor of him in 1832.

5. Nathaniel I. Bowditch, *A History of the Massachusetts General Hospital* (Boston, 1872), 197.

6. *Ibid*, 203.

7. This letter in Holmes's hand was discovered by the author among others from the Autocrat in an uncatalogued folder of correspondence received by Chadwick while he was Librarian of the BML. Chadwick customarily pasted up on heavy sheets letters he thought worth saving from his wide-ranging exchanges, but this was still in its original postmarked envelope, together with this note:

Beverly Farms, Mass.
June 20, 1891.

Dear Dr. Chadwick,

I send you a paper which, if you think its worth while, may be read at the meeting of the

Association of the Alumni. If it *is* to be read, please send it *at once* to Miss
M. W. Macy
28 School St. Room 51
to be type-written and charged to me.—She works often for me and knows my hand well.
It can be read much better from type writing than from my manuscript.
Tell her to make *two* copies and send me one.
Yours very truly,
O. W. Holmes

8. Ware succeeded James Jackson as Hersey Professor of the Theory and Practice of Physic in 1836. Jacob Bigelow and Channing had been professors of materia medica, and of obstetrics and medical jurisprudence, since 1815. Hayward occupied the chair in surgery. The name "passed over in silence" by Holmes was that of John W. Webster, Erving Professor of Chemistry, hanged on August 30, 1850, for the murder of Dr. George Parkman on November 23, 1849, at the Medical School. J. B. S. Jackson came on the faculty as Professor of Pathological Anatomy in 1847, with Holmes. Henry Jacob Bigelow succeeded Hayward as Professor of Surgery in 1849. Storer likewise followed Channing in obstetrics and medical jurisprudence in 1854.

9. Bowditch's appointment as librarian of the MGH is not mentioned by his brother in his *History*. Source for this information is a pamphlet published by the MGH, *Treadwell Library 1858-1958*.

10. Farlow's *History*, 32.

11. From Harvard College Library correspondence folder, Rare Books Department, Countway.

12. Walter Muir Whitehill, *Boston Public Library: A Centennial History* (Cambridge, 1956).

13. *Boston Medical Library. Special Meeting to raise Funds for a New Building, held on November XXIX, MDCCCXCVIII.* Pamphlet published by BML. Pp. 2-3. (Note Chadwick's Roman touch.)

14. Essex County Probate file No. 55630, Salem.

15. *To Work in the Vineyard of Surgery: The Reminiscences of J. Collins Warren (1842-1927)*, Edward D. Churchill, ed. (Cambridge, 1958), 182n-183n.

16. Walter L. Burrage, *A History of the Massachusetts Medical Society* (Boston, 1923), 409-410. Great reliance has been put on Dr. Burrage's work for light shed on the earlier days of the BML and the men active in it. Secretary Burrage penned an interesting epitaph to the Society's library (411):

"It fulfilled one of the functions of a library in promoting friendly relations with similar medical societies and scientific organizations both in this country and abroad. It called the attention of its fellows to the need of the use of books by practitioners of medicine, even though the machinery for providing all the members with reading matter was not perfected as it should have been. It must be remembered that the Massachusetts Medical Society was never affluent. In the early years it was in debt for a large part of the time. It could not afford to hire a librarian whose duty it should be to give his time to the care and distribution of the books of the library. The employment of such an official was the only solution of the problem of how to make the library succeed. Henry Ingersoll Bowditch saw this in 1850, having been brought into close touch with the valuable possessions of the library in the way of records and important papers that had come down from the past. It was necessary for the library to be in a central situation and open for long hours daily under the charge of a permanent regular custodian, in order that it might be useful to a large number and that it might grow in size. These conditions were not met and the books were scattered."

17. Thomas F. Harrington, *The Harvard Medical School. A History, Narrative and Documentary 1782-1905* (New York, 1905), III, 1103-1111. Dr. Har-

rington's *History*, edited by his classmate of 1888, Dr. James G. Mumford, has been liberally drawn upon in the preparation of the BML history.

18. *Ibid.*

19. Farlow's *History*, 35.

20. *Ibid*, 39-40.

3. THE PIED PIPER OF HAMILTON PLACE

1. Surveying the medical literature available to the profession in Boston on one lay or another, Dr. Chadwick found: (1) the medical department of the Boston Public Library contained 9535 volumes in 1876. For ten years it had been growing at an annual rate of about 550, but it was not up to date. It received eighty-seven periodicals regularly. Access to the shelves was by special privilege only; (2) the Athenaeum shelved about five thousand, adding only forty a year. It was obviously inadequate as well as restricted; (3) the Treadwell Library of the MGH, about 3500, was open to non-staff on written application only; (4) Harvard's Boylston Library in Cambridge consisted of 3800, no periodicals; (5) the Harvard Medical School library had around 1800, many of them duplicates, nearly all out of date; (6) rather as a surprise, the library of the Boston Society of Natural History had 12,000 volumes and five hundred journals in the general area of the medical sciences, free to all who applied (J. R. Chadwick, "The Medical Libraries of Boston." First annual report of the Boston Medical Library Association [Cambridge, 1876]).

2. That the "young Turk" viewpoint held sway among the nineteen is further indicated by Chadwick's comment some years later that "a number of us young men decided that the time was ripe for the formation of a medical library as an independent institution, under the control of the profession as a whole, which should bring under one roof the libraries of these two Societies [Observation and Improvement] and such other collections of books as could be secured" (Chadwick, "The Boston Medical Library," *Medical Library and Historical Journal* (1903) I, 127-135). And by H. I. Bowditch, who said at the dedication of the new building on December 3, 1878 that what was needed to put it over was "the young scientific zeal of the present day."

5. Farlow's *History*, 43-44.

4. *Dedication of the New Building and Hall of the Boston Medical Library Association, December 3, 1878.* (Cambridge, 1881), 2-3.

5. Harrington's *History*, II, 867.

6. *BMSJ* CLXVI (December 14, 1911), 932-933.

7. BML 1926 Annual Report, 25-26.

8. Dr. Brigham "took special pains with his handwriting while with Dr. McLaren, taking courses in a business school to perfect it; he developed a skill at bookkeeping and writing records that has stayed with him through life." (Burrage's *History*, 237).

9. Farlow's *History*, 48-49. The movie palace at the dead end of Hamilton Place, Loew's Orpheum until recent years, is on the site of the Music Hall, which was erected in 1852 expressly as a gilded cage to attract Jenny Lind to Boston.

10. Chadwick Papers, Rare Books Department, Countway.

11. *Dedication of the New Building*, 26-27.

12. Fielding H. Garrison, *John Shaw Billings: A Memoir.* (New York, 1915), 213-218.

13. Chadwick Papers.

14. Farlow's *History*, 50.

15. Henry R. Viets, "William Read and His Books," *NEJM* 269 (Sept. 12,

1963), 562-565. The author credits Read with founding in 1861 the Obstetrical Society of Boston, "the oldest special society in American medicine." Ten years after he gave his books to the BML Dr. Read tried, in 1888, to get it to pay him for them; on November 17 the executive committee voted that it was "not in a position to buy them."

16. Farlow's *History,* 53-54.

17. Chadwick Papers.

18. *Dedication of the New Building of the Boston Medical Library, January 12, 1901.* (Boston, 1901), 19.

19. J. S. Billings, "Literature and Institutions," *The American Journal of the Medical Sciences,* October, 1876.

20. The incorporators were O. W. Holmes, H. I. Bowditch, J. R. Chadwick, A. L. Mason, C. P. Putnam, H. P. Bowditch, O. F. Wadsworth, E. Wigglesworth, W. L. Richardson, F. I. Knight, J. C. Warren, R. H. Fitz, J. C. White and T. Dwight. Of the fourteen, twelve are subjects in the *Dictionary of American Biography.*

21. Chadwick Papers. In his *Memoir* (222) Garrison writes that when Billings took over the Surgeon General's Library most of the employes were former hospital stewards "pitchforked" into the job, none educated beyond common schooling, "but as old soldiers they had the dependability and reliability upon which Billings set the highest value. . . Like Emerson's cook who, by dint of cooking the same dinner over and over again, eventually attained perfection, so these old employes, none of them linguists, soon learned the rudimentary techniques of medical bibliography." Chadwick aimed higher, although, curiously enough, his own assistant entered Harvard Medical School with much the same background as Billings's men, from Army hospital stewardship with naught beyond common schooling. The pressing Baltimore work to which Billings refers in this letter was his monumental organization of the Johns Hopkins Hospital.

4. MRS. HOWE'S KITCHEN

1. Farlow's *History,* 58-63.

2. This rarified sanctum was incorporated as a subscription library in 1794. After its quarters on Franklin Street were taken by the city to widen Arch Street, it moved to hired rooms at 20 Essex Street until its purchase of 18 Boylston Place in 1870, which caused its historian to sigh that "there was great loss of dignity in this change, and things were at a very low ebb." A number of shares had been forfeited for nonpayment of assessments. However, things looked up with several bequests and the decision to open the library to annual subscribers who were not shareholders. Samuel S. Shaw, *The Boston Library Society* (Boston, 1895).

3. George Santayana, *Persons and Places* (New York, 1944), 70-71.

4. Chadwick Papers.

5. Farlow's *History,* 67.

6. The remarks of the speakers were published by the BML in a pamphlet, *Dedication of the New Building and Hall of the Boston Medical Library Association, 19 Boylston Place, December 3, 1878.* (Cambridge, 1881). Dr. Holmes included his address, "Medical Libraries," in the 1883 edition of his *Medical Essays.*

7. Rarely during Holmes's presidency from 1875 to 1888 were meetings of the executive committee gathered at the Library, only eleven times in fact. Usually the committee met in Secretary Wadsworth's office at 139 Boylston Street, occasionally at Dr. Wigglesworth's up the street. Of eighty-three meetings, Holmes was present and presided at but twelve.

8. *Transactions of the American Medical Association* XXVIII (1877).
9. *Ibid,* 199-200.
10. Burrage's *History,* 238. After his death Dr. Martin's library on vaccination and smallpox was presented to the BML by his son, Dr. F. C. Martin.
11. Farlow's *History,* 78. Of no recorded practical value at all was the authorization given Chadwick in May 1879 to invite nineteen leading members to be curators in their specialties. Like many such crowned duchies, they collapsed from the weight of protocol and were not even mentioned by the Librarian in his next annual report.
12. A later librarian, Dr. Henry R. Viets, wrote of Frederick Cheever Shattuck in the *Dictionary of American Biography* (New York, 1964) IX, 31: "The picture of the doctor on the back seat of his small Victoria, being driven rapidly behind a pair of fast horses, and without regard for traffic rules through the streets of Boston, is one not easily forgotten. His favorite dachshund and a pile of medical journals were beside him, a cigarette was between his lips, a carnation was in his buttonhole, and a bright waistcoat and a cheery smile for all lent vivid color to the picturesque ensemble."
13. "Report of the Committee on the Directory for Nurses," in BML 1881 Annual Report, 14.
14. *Ibid,* 18. Dr. Shattuck was correct in his prediction. Within a dozen years nurses' directories were functioning in Baltimore, Philadelphia, Brooklyn, Washington, Chicago and San Francisco. (E. J. Forster, "Medical Profession of Suffolk County," in *Professional and Industrial History of Suffolk County* (Boston, 1894) III, 216).
15. "Report of the Committee," 15.
16. Sara E. Parsons, *History of the Massachusetts General Hospital Training School for Nurses* (Boston, 1922), 152-153.
17. Dr. Eugene F. Cordell, the new Librarian of the Medical and Chirurgical Faculty of Maryland, wrote Chadwick from Baltimore on November 21, 1880 that Billings had told him "you had found a source of several hundred dollars revenue in the establishment of a *Nurses' Exchange;*" he wanted to know all about it. (Chadwick Papers.)
18. Farlow's *History,* 86-88.
19. *To Work in the Vineyard of Surgery,* 154.
20. John J. Currier, *History of Newburyport, Massachusetts, 1764-1909* (Newburyport, 1909) II, 556. The "epitaphs" of Hannah F. Gould were published posthumously (or posthumorously.)
21. Holmes's *Memoranda,* 556.
22. BML 1884 Annual Report.
23. *Boston Sunday Globe,* January 24, 1926.
24. Communication to John W. Farlow (Farlow's BML Notes, February 11, 1926).
25. Mrs. Leatherbee hyperbolized the adenoidal contributions (or subtractions) of Dr. Robert W. Hooper, for years a surgeon at the Massachusetts Eye and Ear Infirmary. He and Holmes were classmates at HMS and chums in Paris while studying with Louis. A few days after the funerals of Hooper and another old friend, Dr. Samuel Cabot, OWH wrote James Russell Lowell, on April 29, 1885, "It is as if an autumn wind were tearing away the last leaves all around me." (*Life and Letters of Oliver Wendell Holmes* (Boston, 1896) II, 79.)
26. Burrage's *History,* 239.
27. Santayana's *Persons and Places,* 75-76.
28. November 2, 1885 (Chadwick Papers).
29. Washington, October 3, 1886 (Chadwick Papers). The name of the game is a mystery. Could it have been shuffleboard?

30. Cambridge, April 28, 1882 (Chadwick Papers).
31. W. Fraser Rae, *Columbia and Canada: Notes on the Great Republic and the New Dominion (London, 1877), 173-175.*
32. *Boston Sunday Herald,* March 26, 1899.
33. BML 1887 Annual Report.
34. *BMSJ* CXX (February 7, 1889), 140-144.
35. The proceedings, including Dr. Holmes's address, were published in the *BMSJ,* ibid.

5. THE DIGNITY OF THE PROFESSION AT STAKE

1. BML 1898 Annual Report.
2. BML 1891 Annual Report.
3. BML 1942 Annual Report.
4. *BMSJ* 131:24 (December 13, 1894), 584-590.
5. Dr. Bowditch died in 1892 and left the Library three hundred dollars as a book fund, the first bequest received.
6. *BMSJ* op cit. The cast is in the possession of the Library.
7. James R. Chadwick, "The Boston Medical Library," *Medical Library and Historical Journal* I (1903), 128. Chadwick remarked in this article that the Library was founded by "a number of us young men." *Sic transit gloria juventutis.*
8. The transcript was published by the Library as a pamphlet, *Boston Medical Library. Special Meeting to Raise Funds,* op cit.
9. Chadwick's "The Boston Medical Library."
10. Walter Muir Whitehill, *Boston: A Topographical History* (Cambridge, 1959), 180-183.
11. Farlow's *History,* 114.
12. The pioneer in the treatment of diabetes was eighty-nine when he recalled these events in a letter to Dr. Howard B. Sprague, BML president, dated November 17, 1958 from the Joslin Clinic:

Dear Doctor Sprague:

I would love to give some money to the Boston Medical Library but at present Mrs. Joslin and I must not do it because we are so tied up with Diabetes Foundation, Inc. If we live after 1959, we will be in a more favorable position.

You know how interested I am in the library. When the question came up whether it should be moved from the building downtown to Garrison Street, or to its present location, I was able to furnish the tie vote which I had from Dr. Grace Wolcott which prevented our going to Garrison Street. John Collins Warren was a great help at that time and backed Fred Cotton and me.

Incidentally, when later money was raised for the Library, Fred Cotton and I secured guarantees of $5,000 a year for five years from the younger doctors and eventually every cent of the $25,000 was redeemed.

You see therefore, I really am interested in the Library and regret that I ought not at present to give to it.

Don't trouble to acknowledge this letter.

Sincerely yours,
Elliott P. Joslin

13. *To Work in the Vineyard of Surgery,* 204.
14. BML 1942 Annual Report. How or to what end Henry Holzer and his playmates "ran teets," he did not elaborate.
15. New York, December 12, 1900 (Chadwick Papers).
16. *His wish is gratified by us, his friends,* pronounced Dr. Chadwick, quoting this final verse from an early Holmes poem, "To the Portrait of 'A Lady' in the Athenaeum Gallery."

17. Dr. and Mrs. Fifield's daughter, Mrs. Mary Fifield King, continued to support the Fifield Room after it was adopted by Henry Viets as his office, and left the Library $5000 for its maintenance on her death in 1948.

18. The proceedings were published by the Library in the pamphlet *Dedication of the New Building of the Boston Medical Library,* op cit. Dr. Osler included his address as "Books and Men" in *Aequanimitas,* his collection of medical essays published in 1904.

19. Farlow's *History,* 116-117. New members from outside Suffolk County were formally solicited by a committee on extension of membership, in a circular letter dated March 29, 1901, wherein associate membership at the reduced rate of five dollars was offered as an option.

20. Chadwick Papers.

6. FLOOD IN THE FENWAY

1. BML 1899 Annual Report.
2. Farlow's *History,* 140.
3. Harvard College Librarian's Report, 1901-1902.
4. Farlow's *History,* 151.
5. BML 1904 Annual Report.
6. In 1966 the Cambridge Public Library transferred legal ownership of the Tiedemann Collection to the BML.
7. The Boston Public Library in 1961 offered the BML the balance of its deposit collection, which had been stored at the New England Deposit Library.
8. *BMSJ* CXLIV (March 14, 1901), 264.
9. *Ibid,* 261-262.
10. *Report of a Committee Appointed by the Boston Society for Medical Improvement to Consider Further the Question of the Formation of an Academy of Medicine.* Boston, 1903.
11. James G. Mumford, "The Story of the Boston Society for Medical Improvement," *BMSJ* CXLIV (March 14, 1901), 247-253; Mumford, "Proposed Boston Academy of Medicine," *BMSJ* CXLVI (February 6, 1902), 129-131.
12. Henry R. Viets, biography of James G. Mumford in *Dictionary of American Biography.*
13. The Boston Society for Medical Improvement continued to meet irregularly until 1916, when it all but nominally expired. In 1924 its members voted to disband and turn over the treasury to the BML, designating the income for purchases. Death by corporate dissolution was decreed by the legislature on March 31, 1925. In the same year the BML accepted the remaining funds of the defunct Boston Medical Association.
14. Farlow's *History,* 173.
15. Chadwick Papers. Dr. Chadwick pencilled at the bottom: "This letter relates to a design for a seal for the med. libr. JRC."
16. Walter L. Burrage, obituary of Chadwick in *Transactions of the American Gynecological Society* 31 (1906), 437.
17. Besides naming the periodical room at the rear of the second floor after Chadwick, the Library raised a memorial fund for the purchase of journals in his name and for a tablet for Holmes Hall by R. E. Brooks, the sculptor who did the bust of Dr. Holmes. The Chadwick family loaned the BML a remarkable portrait of him by Wilton Lockwood; this was replaced in 1912 with a copy painted by the artist on subscription. Where the portrait hung, there was the Chadwick Periodical Room, which in 1916 was moved upstairs a flight to take over the so-called Students Room.

18. Farlow's *History*, 180-181.

19. *BMSJ* CLXV (December 14, 1911), 934. Dr. Wadsworth left the BML the balance of his own library on ophthalmology and $10,000, the income to be used for book purchases.

20. BML 1910 and 1911 Annual Reports.

21. BML 1913 Annual Report.

22. John W. Farlow, "The Medical Library and Its Contents," *The Aesculapian* I (December 1908), 9.

23. In a presentation before the Boston Medical History Club on November 18, 1921, Dr. Farlow displayed these curious examples of handicraft and pondered their origin. The Tewksbury skin, given by Mr. J. H. Edmonds, was dated 1883, the year of an inconclusive investigation of the state institution by Governor Benjamin F. Butler. The piratical pouch, contributed by Dr. C. W. Townsend, was said to have been in his family since 1753; Farlow doubted its provenance. Subsequently, in his *Medical Library Notes* for November 5, 1926, he wrote: "Found among Jacob Bigelow's papers a pamphlet 'The Story of George Walton'—the highwayman whose tanned skin BML has."

24. Farlow's "The Medical Library," 8-9.

25. *Ibid*, 9.

26. Farlow's *History*, 105.

27. *Dedication of the New Building of the Boston Medical Library* (1901), 37.

28. Harrington's *History* III, 1157.

29. *To Work in the Vineyard of Surgery*, 208.

30. BML 1913 Annual Report; Farlow's *Medical Library Notes*, April 27, 1913.

31. Farlow's *History*, 186.

32. BML 1913 Annual Report.

33. "When we look about in this building for the room reserved for his use," Farlow noted in his eulogy of Chadwick, "for his desk, for anything pertaining to him alone, we find—nothing. There is no Librarian's room, he had no desk, no closet, no drawer, merely a small wire basket in one corner of a shelf in the cataloguer's room, in which were placed various memoranda, old catalogues, and odds and ends." (BML 1905 Annual Report.)

34. Minutes of the committee on library and finance, March 19 and April 16, 1917.

35. *Ibid*, May 21, 1917.

7. LOVE'S LABOUR'S LOST

1. From a letter to A. Lawrence Lowell in: Joseph C. Aub and Ruth L. Hapgood, *Pioneer in Modern Medicine: David Linn Edsall of Harvard* (Boston, 1970), 214.

2. The summary of the *Journal*'s history is derived from: Joseph Garland, "The Boston Medical and Surgical Journal 1828-1928," *NEJM* 198:1 (Feb. 23, 1928), 1-13, and Burrage's *History*, 359-365. Neither author evidently was aware of the 1919 negotiations with the BML.

3. Frederic T. Lewis Files, in Harvard Medical and Boston Medical Libraries Folder, Rare Books Department, Countway.

4. *Ibid.*

5. *Ibid.*

6. *Ibid*, letter from Lewis to Farlow, December 6, 1919.

7. Farlow, *Medical Library Notes*, December 4 & 5, 1919.

8. *Ibid*, October 21, 1919.

9. The nature of Harvey Cushing's proposition has eluded the author. However, he did lean toward a fused library near the Medical School (and the Brigham) and was friendly with Lewis.
10. Lewis Files.
11. *Ibid.*
12. Dean's Files, Drawer 9, HMS Archives, Rare Books Department, Countway.
13. *Ibid.*
14. Lewis Files.
15. May 27, 1920. Dean's Files.
16. Harvard University Medical Faculty Minutes of Meetings, HMS Archives, Rare Books Department, Countway.
17. Dean's Files.
18. Farlow's *BML Notes,* January 14 & 16, February 1, 1921.
19. *Ibid,* January 17, February 2, 1921.
20. The Thomas Morgan Rotch, Jr., Memorial Infants' Hospital was established in 1914 in memory of the only son of Dr. Thomas Morgan Rotch, first Professor of Pediatrics at HMS, on Shattuck Street, adjacent to the School. The classic marble building merged with the Children's Hospital on the other side of the School, and the vacated structure became the first home of the Harvard School of Public Health. (Jean A. Curran, *Founders of the Harvard School of Public Health* (New York, 1970), 122.)
21. Farlow's *BML Notes,* February 3, 1921.
22. Dean's Files.
23. *Ibid.*
24. Farlow's *BML Notes,* March 1 & 3, 1921.
25. *Ibid,* March 17, 1921.
26. Supposedly Dr. Edsall approached the Carnegie Corporation, not the Foundation.
27. Lewis Files.
28. *Ibid,* (manuscript draft).
29. *Ibid.*
30. Dean's Files.
31. Hugh Hawkins, biography of Lowell, *Dictionary of American Biography,* Supplement 3.
32. Farlow's *BML Notes,* April 12, 1921.
33. *Ibid,* April 28, May 28, December 27, 1921; January 7, 1922.
34. Lewis Files. Lewis to Joslin, January 13, 1923.
35. *Ibid,* Joslin to Lewis, January 16, 1923.

8. TOO MUCH TOO SOON, TOO LITTLE TOO LATE

1. Farlow's *BML Notes,* June 4, 1919.
2. BML 1919 Annual Report. Colonel Garrison replaced Osler as the Library's sole honorary member. In 1939, not long before his death, Cushing was elected the first honorary Fellow in several years.
3. "The anti-vivisectionists have openly protested against the prostitution of Red Cross funds for animal experimentation under such 'celebrated vivisectionists' as Crile, Cannon, and myself." Cushing's diary, May 16, 1918. (John F. Fulton, *Harvey Cushing–A Biography.* Springfield, Ill. 1946, 428.)
4. Farlow's *BML Notes,* February 1, 1927.
5. *Celebration of the Fiftieth Anniversary of the Boston Medical Library, January 19, 1926.* BML, 14.

6. Farlow's *BML Notes,* January 28, 1920; June 25, 1921.
7. *Ibid,* January 9, 1928; April 26, 27, 29, May 2, 1927; May 21, 1920.
8. *Ibid,* November 28, 1919.
9. *BMSJ* 187:22 (Nov. 30, 1922), 810.
10. Farlow's *BML Notes,* January 27, 1923; November 7, 1925.
11. *Ibid,* January 13, 1920; January 5, 1923.
12. BML 1922 Annual Report. (The subject did not recur.)
13. W. B. McDaniel, "James Francis Ballard 1878-1955" (obituary), *Bulletin of the Medical Library Association* 44:1 (1956), 93.
14. Obituary of Channing Frothingham, *New York Times,* August 13, 1959.
15. Farlow's *BML Notes,* May 16, 1927.
16. BML 1947 Annual Report.
17. Farlow's *BML Notes,* December 14 and 15, 1927.
18. BML 1927 Annual Report.
19. *Ibid.*
20. *Ibid.*
21. *Ibid.*
22. BML 1929 Annual Report.
23. Fulton, *op cit,* 584-585.
24. *Harvard Medical Alumni Bulletin* 3 (October 1928), 4-6.
25. Colonel Garrison, on his retirement from the Army and its Medical Library in May 1930, was immediately appointed Librarian of the Welch Medical Library at Johns Hopkins.
26. Frederic T. Lewis files, *op cit.*
27. *Ibid,* Lowell to Lewis, May 3, 1930.
28. *Ibid,* Lewis to Hale, May 10, 1930.
29. *Ibid,* Hale to Lewis, May 12, 1930.
30. *Ibid,* Lewis to Cushing, May 10, 1930.
31. *Ibid,* Cushing to Lewis, May 12, 1930.
32. The *Synopsis of the Practice of Preventive Medicine* was published by the Harvard University Press in 1929, edited by Dr. Shields Warren, with an introduction by Dr. Edsall, as a handbook based on preventive work in the various departments of the Medical School. When it appeared, wrote the Dean's close friend and biographer, the late Dr. Joseph C. Aub, "the Harvard Medical School blushed a collective crimson. Some departments were faultlessly represented, but others who had made a rather hasty response to the original questionnaire saw their outlines appear in print without their having had the opportunity of revising the proofs, and at least one department which had made no response at all found that the chapter attributed to it made a travesty of fifteen years of medical progress. Some departments had simply been omitted." (Aub's *Edsall,* 306.)
33. On February 18, 1929, six months before Dr. Prince's death on August 31, the executive committee voted, without explanation in the minutes and on motion of Dr. Painter, to rescind the action of an earlier committee in 1905 in naming the periodical room after an earlier librarian, James Read Chadwick.

9. DOLDRUMS

1. Ballard compiled *A Catalogue of the Medieval and Renaissance Incunabula in the Boston Medical Library* (Boston 1944) in which he stated erroneously (116) that Dr. Homans bought the *Fasciculus medicinae* at auction in 1906, an impossibility since Homans died in 1903. The Hunt auction was held in Boston in October 1893 (Farlow's *History,* 102). The cut-off date for

incunabula has been variously established. *Webster's Second International Dictionary* (1935) defines them as works printed before 1500; the *Third International* (1965) favors 1501.

2. Ballard described several copies of works by Arnoldus de Villa Nova in his *Catalogue* (op cit), none published in 1491, however. In fact, there is no evidence of publication by Arnoldus in 1491. The date given in the annual report may be a misprint, of course. The identity of Dr. Bullard's first incunable remains a mystery.

3. James F. Ballard, *A Catalogue of Medical Incunabula Contained in The William Norton Bullard Loan Collection Deposited in the Boston Medical Library* (Boston, 1929).

4. *Ibid,* vii-viii.

5. Personal communication.

6. *The New England Journal of Medicine* 204:20 (May 14, 1931), 1007:

"During the past years, Dr. Bullard and Mr. Ballard of the Boston Medical Library worked together in assembling a Library such as might have been gathered for reference by large independent medical institutions in the 15th century."

7. BML Annual Report in Abstract. *NEJM* 210:9 (March 1, 1934), 492-494.

8. Frederic A. Washburn, M.D. *The Massachusetts General Hospital: Its Development, 1900-1935* (Boston, 1939), 76.

9. BML correspondence relating to the Harvard books, *op cit.*

10. *Ibid.*

11. BML 1934 Annual Report.

12. BML correspondence, *op cit,* Lincoln Davis to George R. Minot.

13. Trustees' minutes, March 20, 1939.

14. BML 1932 Annual Report.

15. BML 1935 Annual Report. Dr. Davis mistakenly identified Mrs. Sargent as Dr. Holmes's sister and as Mrs. Amelia Jackson Sargent; her maiden name was Amelia Jackson Holmes.

16. BML 1932 Annual Report.

17. BML 1940 Annual Report.

18. BML 1937-1938 Annual Reports.

19. Obituary of John W. Farlow in *Bulletin of the Medical Library Association* 26:1 (1937), 102-103.

20. Dr. Viets's 1930 account was the first since Dr. Samuel Abbott Green's *History of Medicine in Massachusetts* (Boston, 1881), based on his centennial address before the Massachusetts Medical Society on June 7, 1881.

21. Benjamin Spector, "Henry Rouse Viets, 1890-1969: Neurologist, Medical Historian, Librarian." *Bulletin of the History of Medicine* XLIV:2 (March-April, 1970), 173-175.

22. BML 1938 Annual Report.

23. BML 1935 Annual Report.

24. Executive committee minutes, July 17 and October 26, 1936.

25. Trustees' minutes, March 20, 1939.

26. BML 1940 Annual Report.

27. Executive committee minutes, July 17, 1936.

10. MODERNISM'S GRIM TOUCH

1. Thomas P. Fleming, *A Factual Survey of Medical Libraries in Boston* (New York, 1941), 15-16.

2. *Ibid,* 33.

3. Probably most comparable was the library of the College of Physicians of

Philadelphia. Between 1920 and 1940 circulation at the BML rose from 25,133 to 41,857, at Philadelphia from 22,704 to 58,899. At the Kings County Medical Society in Brooklyn it leaped from 13,704 in 1922 to 81,421 in 1940. (*Ibid*, 3.)

4. *Ibid*, 15.
5. Obituary of David Cheever, *NEJM* 253:11 (September 15, 1955), 482-483.
6. BML 1941 Annual Report.
7. To the extent that they could, Viets wrote in the BML 1946 Annual Report, European booksellers had saved periodicals during the war, so that some back numbers were available.
8. BML 1943 Annual Report.
9. BML 1942 Annual Report.
10. James F. Ballard, "Some Problems in the Administration of a Medical Library" (presented at the annual meeting of the Medical Library Association, Atlantic City, N.J., June 22-23, 1914). *Bulletin of the Medical Library Association* 4:3 (January 1915), 41.
11. W. B. McDaniel 2nd, obituary of Ballard, *op cit.*
12. *Ibid.*
13. *Ibid.*
14. *Ibid.*
15. More than 1000 copies of the third edition were sold. The old classification still applies to old and newly acquired BML and Harvard books published before 1950. All published since 1950 are classified according to the system of the National Library of Medicine.
16. BML 1944 Annual Report.
17. Trustees' minutes, April 16, 1945.
18. *Ibid*, March 16, April 21, 1942; BML 1942 Annual Report.
19. BML 1944 Annual Report.
20. Trustees' minutes, November 20, 1944, April 16, October 15, November 19, 1945; BML 1945 Annual Report.
21. Trustees' minutes, April 16, 1945.
22. BML 1945 Annual Report.
23. Trustees' minutes, February 17, 1947.
24. BML 1946 Annual Report.
25. Miss Binderup returned, as Assistant Librarian for Reference Services in the Countway.
26. Trustees' minutes, April 25, 1949. Miss Sanda Countway, whose gift made possible the Francis A. Countway Library of Medicine in memory of her brother, contributed one million dollars in 1958 to erect the Science Museum's central building.
27. BML 1950 & 1951 annual reports.
28. Jean Burton, *Lydia Pinkham Is Her Name* (New York, 1949); *JAMA* 117:26 (December 27, 1941), 2269-2270.
29. BML 1950 Annual Report.
30. Trustees' minutes, October 10, 1951.
31. BML 1949 Annual Report.
32. BML 1952 Annual Report.
33. "Report to the Special Committee of the Board of Trustees, Boston Medical Library, submitted by Anderson and Beckwith, Architects, 2 May 1952."
34. BML 1952 Annual Report.
35. "Fund-Raising Survey Report made for Boston Medical Library, Boston, Massachusetts," by Marts & Lundy, Inc.
36. McDaniel, *op cit.*
37. Henry R. Viets, obituary of James Francis Ballard (signed H.R.V.), *NEJM* 252:24 (June 16, 1955), 1052-1053.

38. McDaniel, *op cit.*
39. Trustees' minutes, September 8, 1954.

11. LOVE'S LABOUR'S RETRIEVED

1. *New and Nonofficial Remedies* (1953), 529, 575, 534.
2. Reports of the Council on Pharmacy and Chemistry, *JAMA* XLIV:22 (June 3, 1905), 1790-1792; XLV:1 (July 1, 1905), 55; XLV:19 (November 4, 1905), 1422.
3. *Ibid,* LIII:7 (August 14, 1909), 569-570.
4. *Ibid,* LXII:19 (May, 1914), 1492-1493.
5. *Ibid,* LXIX:21 (November 24, 1917), 1815-1816.
6. *Nostrums and Quackery,* Volume II. Arthur J. Cramp, M.D., ed. (AMA, Chicago, 1921), 491-492.
7. The minutes of Dr. Berry's first meeting with the Overseers' Visiting Committee on April 28, 1950: noted: "The necessity for rearrangement and expansion of existing library facilities was made clear." (*Bibliotheca Medica: Physician for Tomorrow,* David McCord, ed. (Harvard, 1966), 7).
8. Sources on Francis Countway: Robert W. Lovett, "Francis A. Countway and 'The Lever Way.' " *Harvard Library Bulletin* XVIII:1 (January 1970), 84-93; "Mr. Countway Takes the Job," *Fortune* XXII:5 (November 1940), 94-120.
9. Sister Mary Rosa, quoted in an interview in *The Chelsea Record,* May 28, 1965, in *Bibliotheca Medica,* op cit, 16.
10. George Packer Berry in *ibid,* 210.
11. C. Sidney Burwell, "The Harvard Medical Library: The Problem and the Plan." *Harvard Medical Alumni Bulletin* (February 1959).
12. "Of Libraries and Their Relations," editorial, *NEJM* 260:3 (January 15, 1959), 139-140.
13. Trustees' minutes, January 21, 1959.
14. In 1964 Dr. Soutter was appointed the first dean of the "paper" University of Massachusetts Medical School.
15. Charles H. Bradford, M.D., "Supplementary Considerations for Guidance in Planning Projected Collaborative Medical Library" (unsigned), in Trustees' minutes, February 17, 1959.
16. *The Boston Medical Library committee* (and interests represented): Howard B. Sprague, chairman, BML; Earle M. Chapman, BML; Mr. Charles C. Colby III, BML; Grant V. Rodkey, Allen Fund, BML; John W. Norcross, Lahey Room, BML; Mr. Robert L. Bradford, BML attorney; Joseph Garland, *NEJM*; Carl Bearse, Mass. Medical Society; Charles C. Lund, MMS; Lamar Soutter, BU Medical School; Joseph M. Hayman, Jr., Tufts Medical School; Lawrence R. Dame, physicians outside the Boston area.

The Harvard Medical School Committee: Richard Warren, chairman; George Packer Berry, Dean; C. Sidney Burwell; Dale G. Friend; Mr. Ralph T. Esterquest; Mr. Oscar M. Shaw, attorney; Mr. Douglas W. Bryant, Harvard Librarian; Mr. Paul H. Buck, Director of University Libraries.

17. *BMQ* 10:1 (March 1959), 23-24.
18. "A Tide in the Affairs—" editorial, *NEJM* 260:20 (May 14, 1959), 1040-1041.
19. Trustees' minutes, June 24, 1959.
20. "A Note on the Boston Medical Library" editorial, *BMQ* 10:2 (June 1959), 62.
21. "Boston Medical Library—A Year of Decision" editorial, *NEJM* 261:26 (December 24, 1959), 1345-1346; Walter G. Phippen, "An Adventure in Co-Operation," *ibid,* 1347-1348.

22. The first three BML members of the Joint Library Committee were Howard B. Sprague, Franz J. Ingelfinger and David P. Boyd; for HMS, George Packer Berry, Dale G. Friend and Douglas W. Bryant. Their inaugural meeting was on December 15, 1964.

12. UNION

1. Howard B. Sprague, "President's Report at the Annual Meeting of the Fellows of the Boston Medical Library, April 17, 1967." *Harvard Library Bulletin* XV:4 (October 1967), 417.
2. *Building Program for the New Francis A. Countway Library of Medicine of the Harvard Medical School and the Boston Medical Library.* Working Edition, revised March 1961.
3. George Packer Berry, "To the Members of the Visiting Committee," subject: The Francis A. Countway Library of Medicine. February 23, 1960. (mimeographed)
4. *Building Program,* op cit.
5. Berry, *op cit.*
6. Ralph T. Esterquest, "The Francis A. Countway Library of Medicine: Its Facilities, Resources and Services" (presented at the annual meeting of the Massachusetts Medical Society, May 22, 1962). *Tufts Medical Alumni Bulletin* (November 1962).
7. *Bibliotheca Medica,* op cit, xvii.
8. *Ibid,* 132.
9. *Ibid,* 243.
10. *Ibid,* 217.
11. Ann T. Curran, "The Mechanization of the Serial Records for the Moving and Merging of the Boston Medical and Harvard Medical Serials." *Library Resources and Technical Services* 10:3 (summer 1966), 362.
12. Berry, *op cit.*
13. Trustees' minutes, March 18, 1959.
14. Henry R. Viets, "From the Curator's Notebook: An Errant Incunable." *NEJM* 273:4 (July 22, 1965), 224-225.
15. Ralph T. Esterquest, "The Program of the Francis A. Countway Library of Medicine" (presented at the annual meeting of the Medical Library Association, Boston, June 7, 1966). *Bulletin of the Medical Library Assocation* 55:1 (January 1967), 40.
16. The entire proceedings of the dedication of the Countway Library, including texts of addresses, were published in *Bibliotheca Medica.*
17. *Bibliotheca Medica,* op cit, 208-210.
18. *Ibid,* 230.
19. Berry, *op cit.*
20. Esterquest, "The Program," *op cit,* 40-41.
21. Sprague, *op cit,* 414.
22. Joseph Garland, *A Time for Remembering* (*NEJM,* Boston, 1972), 193.
23. In 1966 the endowment was enlarged by $30,000 designated for book purchases by the late Dr. Annie E. Taft, who died in Narberth, Pa., in 1964. She had visited the BML frequently some years earlier and was remembered by Charles Colby as "a very kind and appreciative person."
24. Harold Bloomquist, "Ralph T. Esterquest, 1912-1968." *Harvard Medical Alumni Bulletin* 43:1 (fall 1968), 42-43.
25. The ground-floor office of the Associate Librarian for BML Services is designated the Wadsworth Memorial Room, another carry-over from 8 The Fenway.

26. Oliver Wendell Holmes, "Dedicatory Address," in *Dedication of the New Building and Hall of the Boston Medical Library Association,* op cit, 14-15.

27. Harold Bloomquist, memorandum dated August 15, 1974.

Index